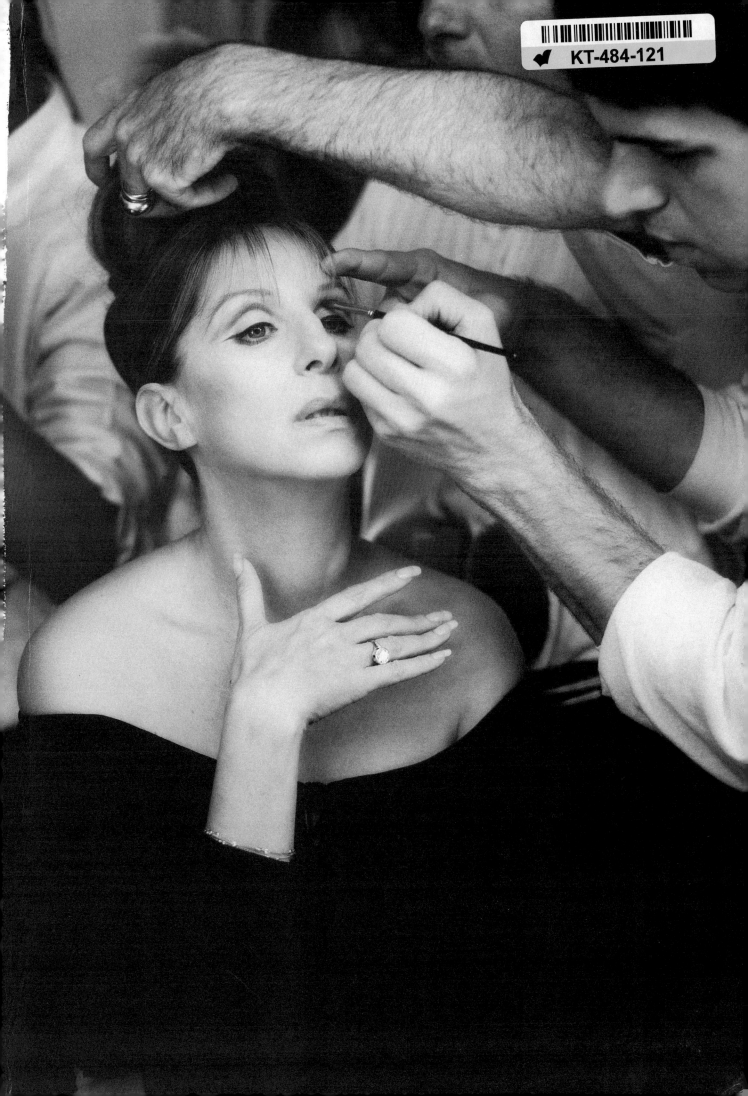

Books by Kevyn Aucoin

The Art of Makeup
Making Faces
Face Forward

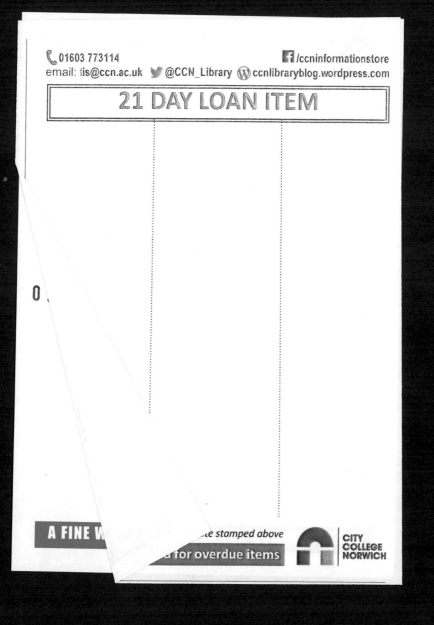

Kevyn Aucoin a beautiful life

the success, struggles, and beauty secrets of a legendary makeup artist

Written by Kerry Diamond   Creative direction by Eric Sakas
Art direction by Julian Peploe   Co-creative direction by Sandra Collado
All makeup by Kevyn Aucoin

ATRIA BOOKS

New York   London   Toronto   Sydney

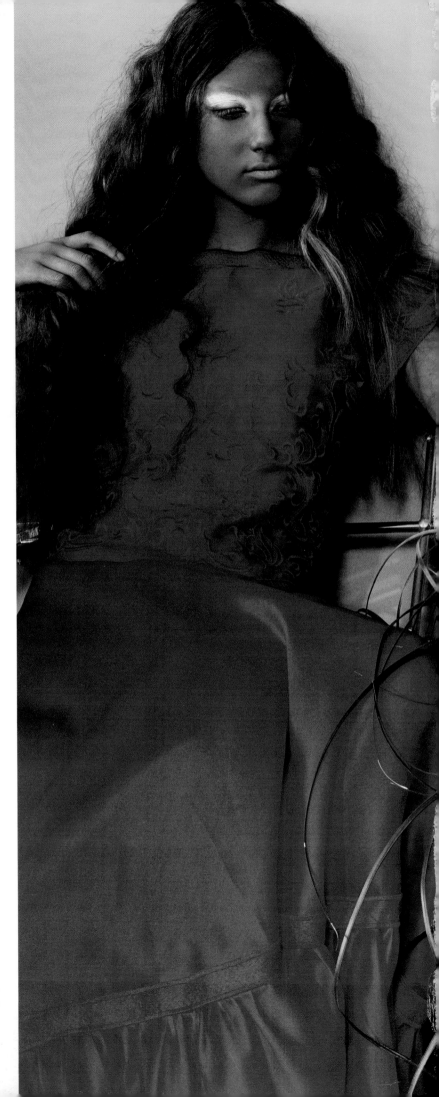

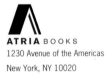

ATRIA BOOKS

1230 Avenue of the Americas

New York, NY 10020

ISBN: 0-7434-5642-4

0-7432-3583-5 (Pbk)

First Atria Books trade paperback edition October 2004

10 9 8 7 6 5 4 3 2 1

ATRIA BOOKS is a trademark of Simon & Schuster, Inc.

Design by Julian Peploe

Manufactured in the United States of America

For information regarding special discounts for bulk purchases,
please contact Simon & Schuster Special Sales
at 1-800-456-6798 or business@simonandschuster.com

Lyrics from "Taxi Ride" by Tori Amos, appearing on page 153,
copyright © 2002, by Sony Music Entertainment, Inc.

Photo by Steven Klein © 1999 Italian *Vogue*
Courtesy of Condé Nast Publications Inc.

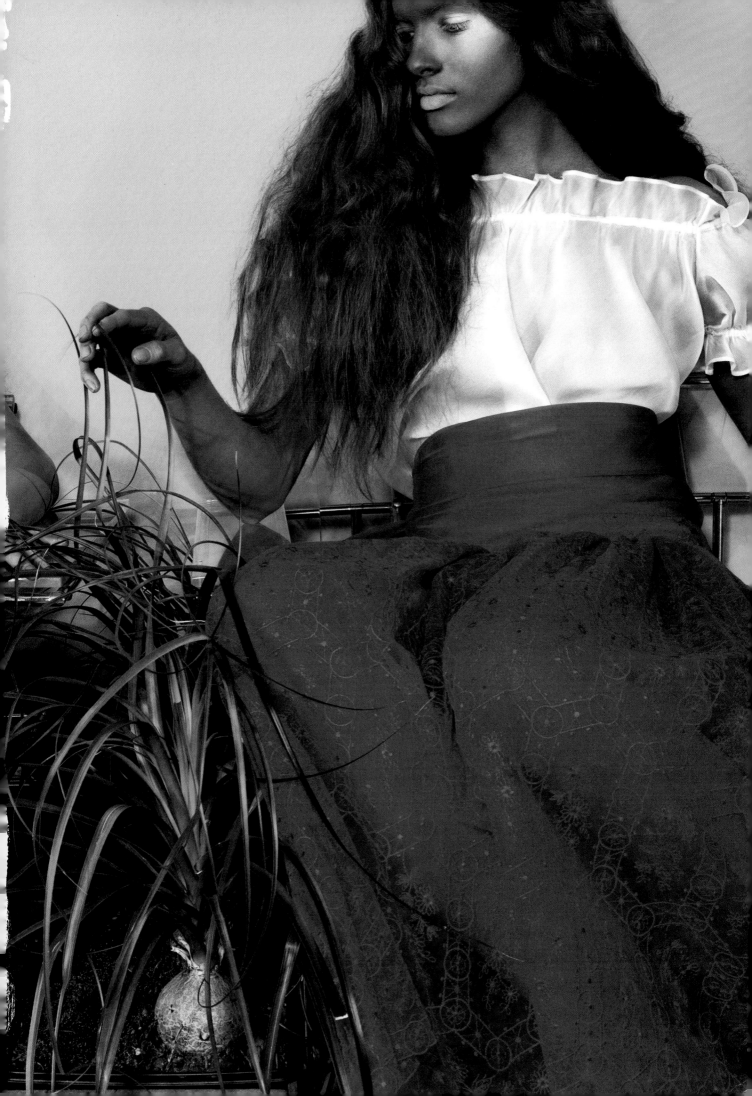

LAY YOUR HEAD UPON THE SEASHORE
LAY YOUR HEAD UPON THE SAND
LISTEN FOR THE WAVE WITHIN YOU
LISTEN NOW AND UNDERSTAND

KNOW THE MERCY OF THE WATER
KNOW THE SAFETY OF THE DEEP
FIND THE COMFORT WE'RE ALL BORN WITH
HEAR THE VOICE THAT GIVES YOU PEACE

—KEVYN AUCOIN

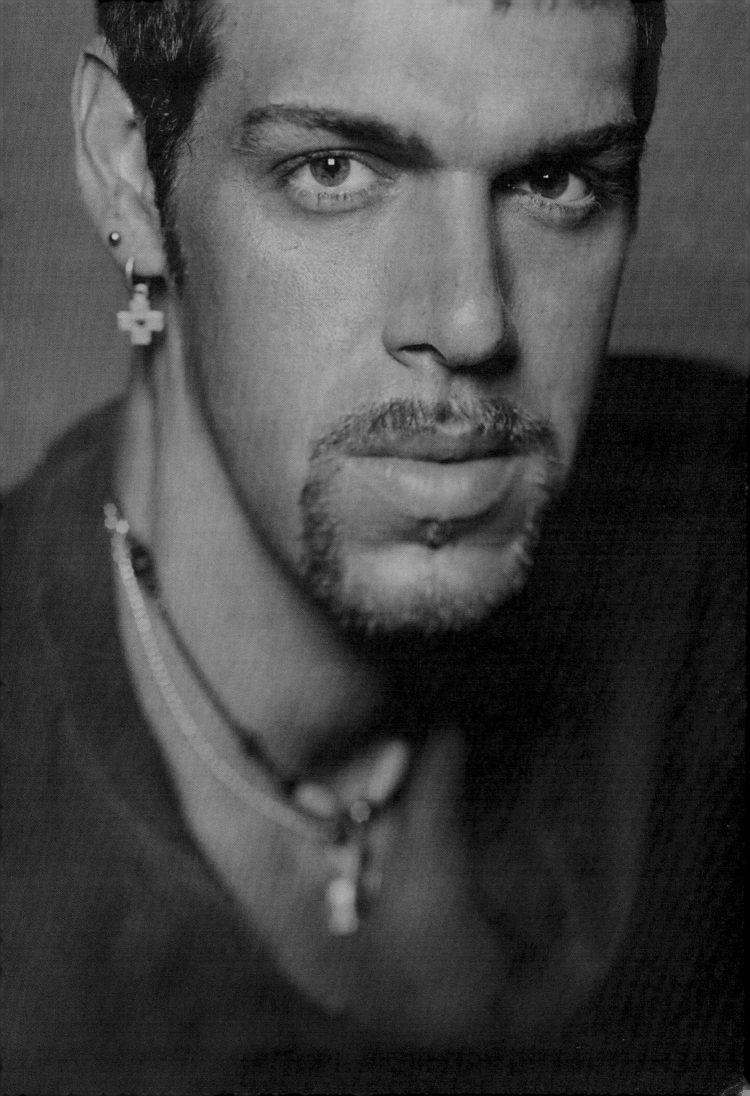

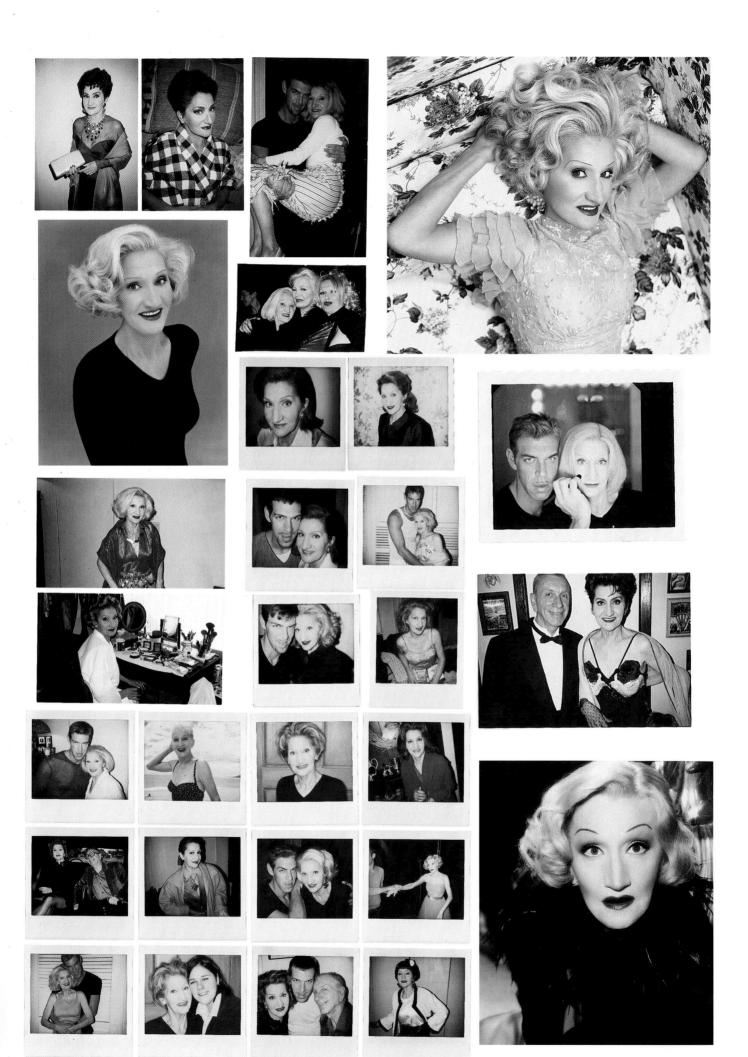

This book is dedicated to the memory of Kevyn's beloved moma, Thelma Aucoin.

1934–2002

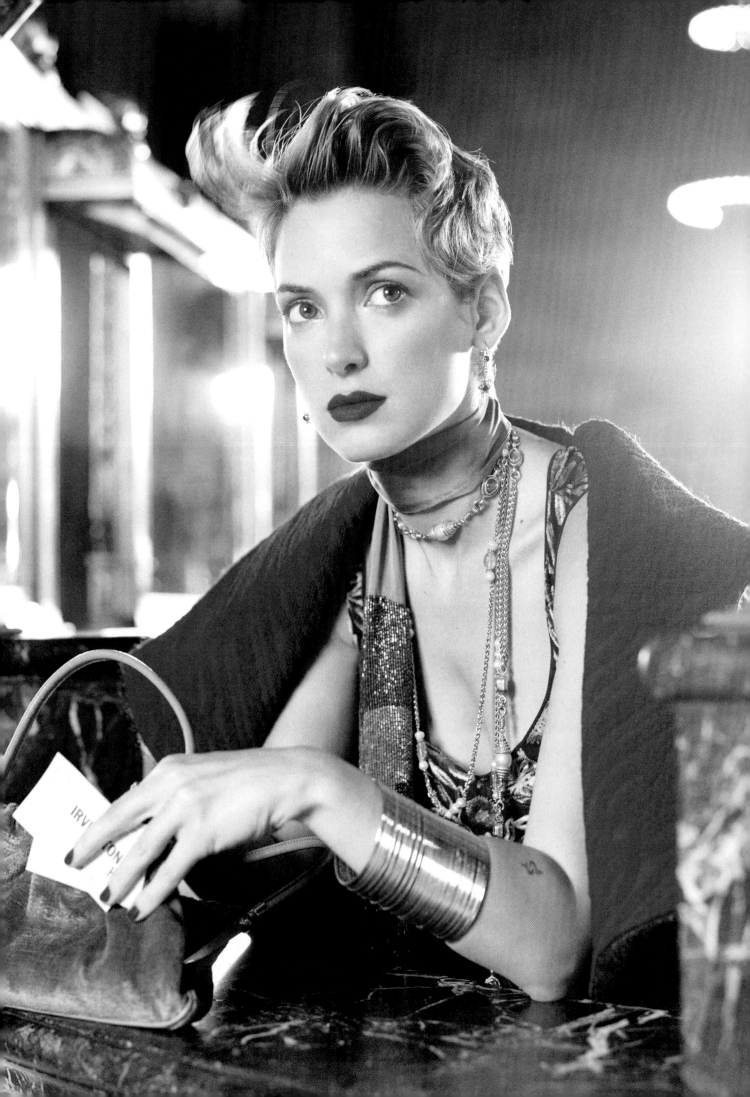

ACKNOWLEDGMENTS

The *Beautiful Life* team would like to thank the following people for their assistance and support:

The Aucoin family, Paul Abrantes, Julie Agrati, Zaki Amin, Taylor Anderton, Ellen Arcuri, Rebecca Arnold, Erik Asla, Gena Avery, Richard Baccari, Ji Baek, Glenda Bailey, Ivan Bart, Michelle Bega, Nancy Behrman, Zana Benson, Cindi Berger, Jenna Berkowitz, Ed Burstell, Lina Bey, Wayde Binder, Evyn Block, Pete Born, Sean Byrnes, Anthony Carro, Chad Carr, Kathryn Coffman, Patti Cohen, Ricardo Collado, Stephanie Cone, Sarah Corrao, Anna Crean, Kim Creighton, Camilla de Crespigny, Judith Curr, Sarah Dawes, Debbie Deuble, Sheryl Diamond, John Diamond, Kathy Djonlich, Paige Dorian, Elaine Drepot, Sabrina Dupre, Marcy Engelman, Michael Falco, John Firestone, Robert Forrest, Melissa Foss, Karen Gerwin, Suzanne Gluck, Arlu Gomez, Rhonda Graam, Erica Gray, Lizzy Grubman, Alana Hall, Terri Harris, Breanne Heldman, Greer Hendricks, Austin Higgins, Jaclyn Holland, Steve Huvane, June Jacobs, Billy Jim, Jim Johnson, Karin Kato, Victoria Kirby, Lorraine Krich, Lynn LaMoine, Elizabeth Lamont, Cary Leitzes, Cindy Lewis, Michael Long, Rachel Low, Wayne Lukas, Fern Mallis, Jessica Matlin, Melissa McCarthy, Newell McNair, Jaime Mendoza, Nathalie Moar, Leigh Montville, Kristin Moses, Susan Murphy, Troy Nankin, Suzanne O'Neill, Janet Ozzard, Ricky Pannell, Casey Patterson, Becky Pentland, Kristin Perrotta, Alex Peruzzi, Jessica Poblete, Mia Roberts Stern, Jed Root, Brett Ross, David Ryan, Laura Saio, Valerie Salembier, Karen Samfilippo, Lindsay Scott, Terry Sims, Lindsey Simmen, Kim Skalecki, Lauren Smith, Liz Smith, Michael Stier, Troy Surratt, Jacquie Tractenberg, Kate Trimble, Cara Tripicchio, Jenny Turner, Shannon Urbon, Chie Ushio, Brenda Ventura, Samantha Walsh, Jason Weisenfeld, Linda Wells, Sam Wilson, and John Witherspoon.

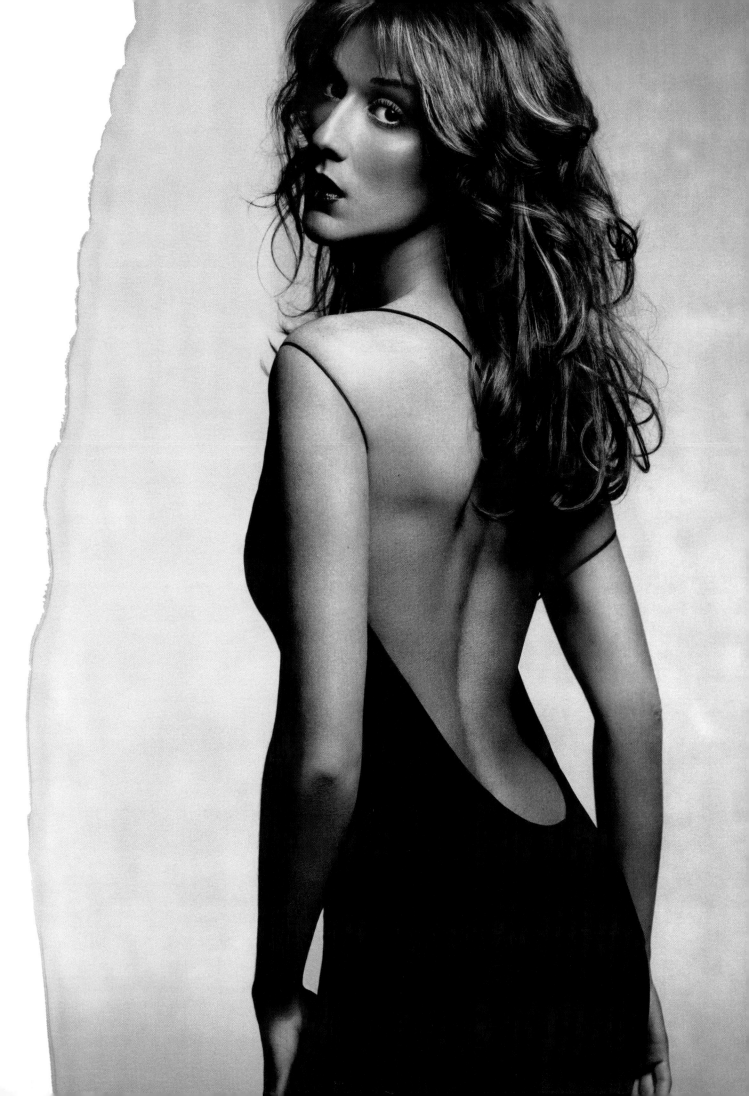

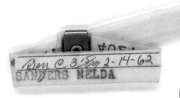

contents

Opposite: Celine Dion by Kevyn Aucoin.   Above: Kevyn's baby bracelet.

Kevyn
Aucoin
a beautiful life

introductions

When I conjure Kevyn, I see his hands first. His impossibly big hands. The long fingers and thick knuckles. I always marveled at how those giant hands were able to work with such grace and precision. They would encompass my face, and with a few brusque touches I would be transformed. Sometimes into a postmodern woman, sometimes into a sultry charcoal-eyed vixen, sometimes into a man or an icon from another era, but mostly just a better version of myself. He would lay me down on the floor like a canvas, the way Jackson Pollock would, and begin. As I lay there, we would listen to music and talk about our lives in a way that we wouldn't when we were out to dinner or at a party. We would talk about childhood and lovers or the letdowns of life. He would tell me obscene jokes and scream his loud, throaty laugh.

He was always striving toward a deeper understanding of things. He wanted to be clearer, better, stronger all the time. Sometimes he would feel set back, but he would persevere, and always with great humor.

He was good to his friends. He knew what love was and how to show it, even though deep down he didn't always feel worthy of it himself. He was decent and generous, and he redefined fashion makeup. I will forever miss him on those big days when he would have been there to get me ready. But I will still hear him call me "monkey," and I will still hear him guffawing. I will still hear him monopolize the stereo at a photo shoot, taking off whatever trendy music is playing and putting on some of his white-girl folk music. I will still see him strip down to a tank top when it is snowing outside. And I will forever see those hands, their strength and assuredness and fragility and beauty. All that Kevyn was and always will be.

Gwyneth Paltrow

kevyn aucoin: a beautiful life

Photo by Michael Thompson © 1997 French *Vogue*. Courtesy of Condé Nast Publications Inc.

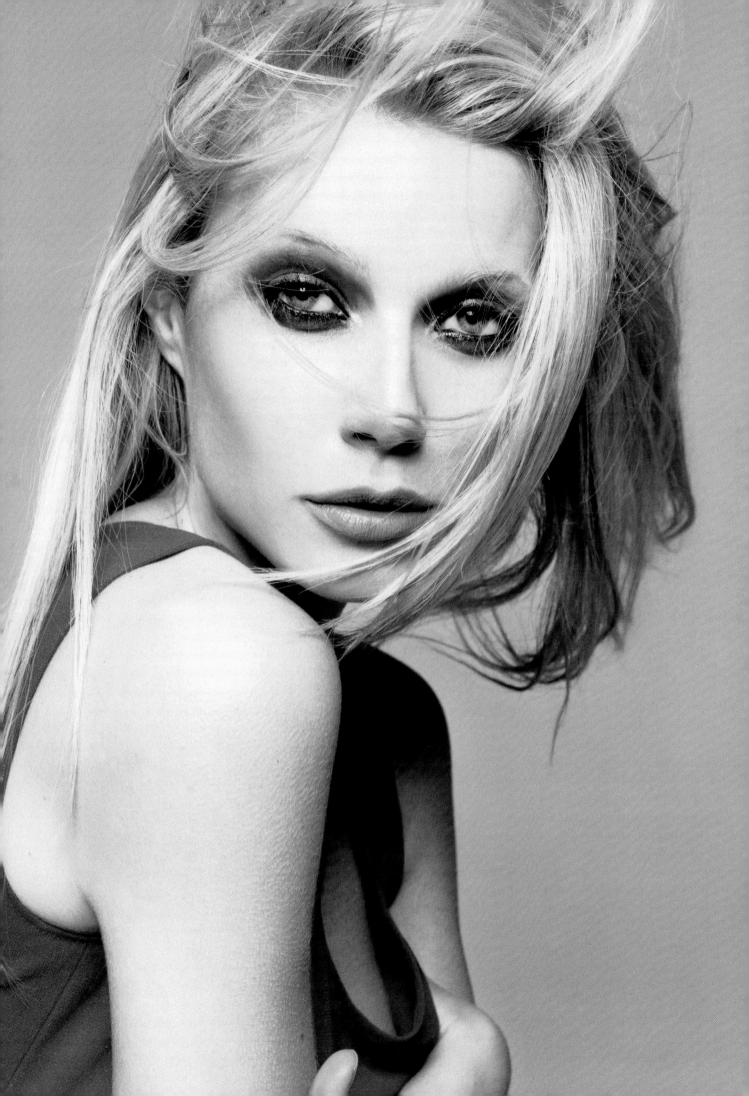

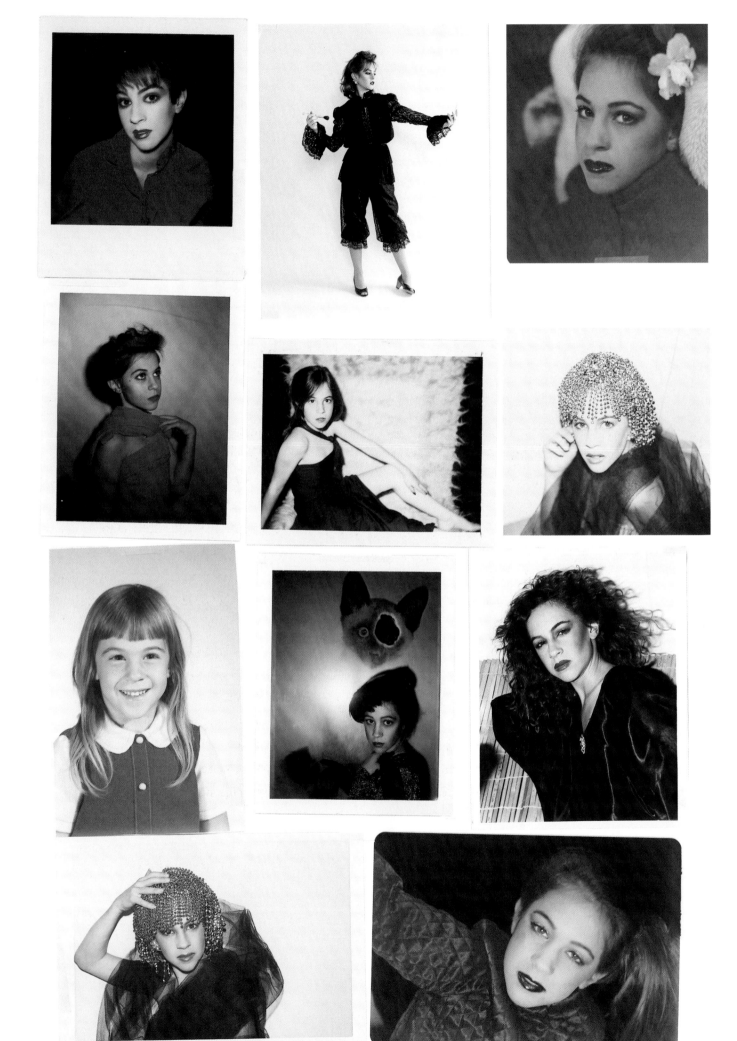

I'm Kevyn's sister, his very first muse, and the mother of his beloved niece Samantha, whom he considered his daughter. When I was just a kid, and I would visit Kevyn at his tiny apartment in our hometown of Lafayette, Louisiana, he always wanted to do my makeup and take pictures of me. You never just hung out and slept at Kevyn's place. You threw something on, you were in front of the camera, and he did this and that.

Later, he always told people it was so torturous for me, but I don't remember it that way. I'd always have to lie on the floor or the bed, because that's how Kevyn liked to do your makeup. His hand was so big it covered my entire head. Posing for him wasn't hard work. It was like, "Just stand there." For me, it was fun because I got to hang out with my big brother, and I didn't have to be home, listening to my parents.

Besides, what else was I going to do? We didn't have a lot of money, so we weren't going to the movies or going roller-skating. Kevyn was the thing. He'd always say, "We're gonna go to New York, and you can be a model." Of course, I never grew past five-foot-two!

Everyone always asks me what Kevyn was like as a kid. The truth is, he never changed. Once, when I was visiting in New York, I mentioned that some people were staring at him. He was like, "Why? I'm a nobody." But Kevyn was somebody. He was a very strong, spirited person who shared everything he had with his family, his friends, even strangers. He wanted people to understand that no matter what obstacles were put in their way, hard work and perseverance could help them achieve what they wanted out of life. Please know that Kevyn might be gone, but his spirit and love will never leave us.

Carla Aucoin Hoffkins

I've been mourning Kevyn more than I expected to. When I told Oprah what I was going through, she said, "Well, Tina, he was always in your face." She was absolutely right. When someone gets that close to you and is studying your features and staring into your eyes, you really get to know him. We had a true connection from the very first time we worked together. I had wanted to do my own makeup for the photo shoot, but I was persuaded to use a professional artist. When I walked into the studio, there was this tall, skinny boy wearing a wool cap. Even before he did my makeup, there was a twinkle in his eye. We didn't talk as he got started. He was in my face, breathing on me, and I was breathing on him. All of a sudden, we made eye contact, and we both just burst out laughing. That broke the ice, and we became friends.

From that moment on, no one did my makeup except for Kevyn. We had so much fun, and it was like a reunion every time we saw each other. He was always there for me. I trusted him completely, and I knew he would take care of me when I was in his hands. I always watched him carefully so that I could try his techniques when I had to do my own makeup. He was so patient, and he would go step by step. He was such a natural, and he was really proud of the fact that he had taught himself how to do makeup.

Most makeup artists and photographers take a lifetime to become the best that they can be, but Kevyn got there by the age of forty. His life was too short, but I honestly don't think he could have topped himself. He had achieved everything he set out to do and more.

Shortly after Kevyn passed away, a companion of mine was clearing some papers from his desk when a letter from Kevyn suddenly fell to the ground. At the end of the letter, he had written, "And by the way, do take care of my friend," referring to me. We were both chilled and felt Kevyn's presence in the room. Perhaps when he wrote the letter he had known on some level that he would be leaving this earth and how deeply it would affect me. He was a true friend, and I hope he felt that I took care of him, just as he wanted me looked after.

I can't imagine what it will be like to work with someone else. It's going to be quite a task. For me, there will never be another Kevyn.

Tina Turner

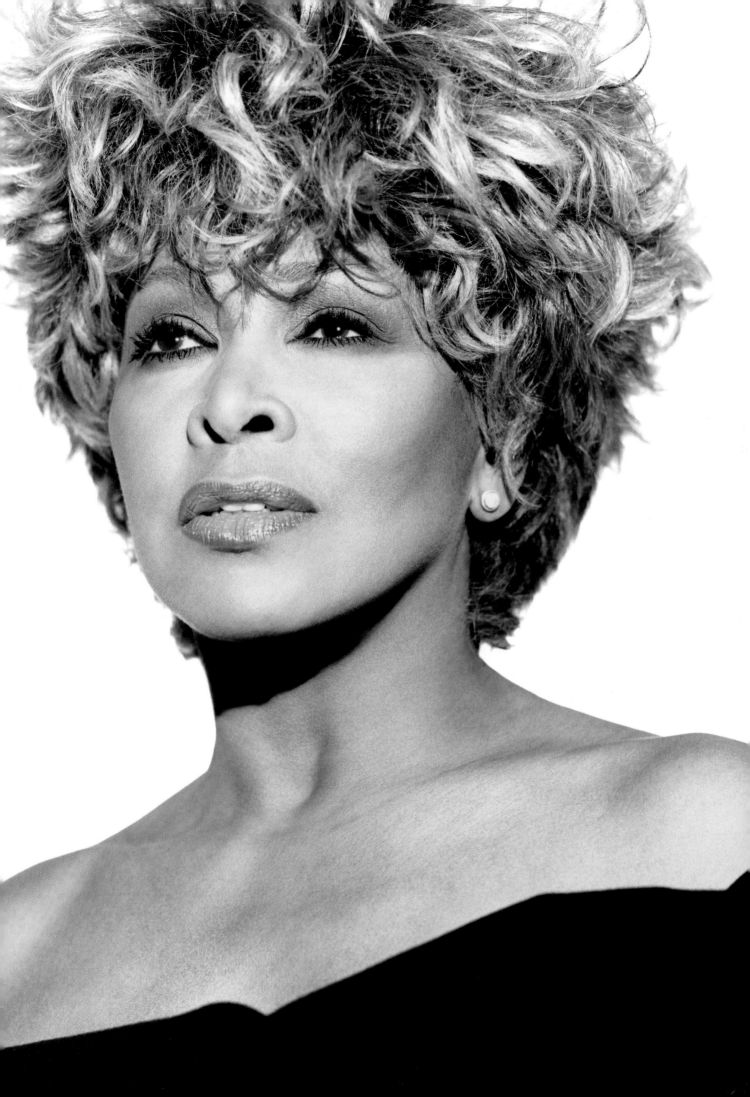

I have often heard it said of Kevyn that he was larger than life. Now, some people would say that this was because of his size, but it wasn't. It was because of his ability to magnify everything. Every situation, experience, and emotion that life made available to him, Kevyn embraced.

Relating to any makeup artist is always an incredibly intimate experience. There is no shying away from the closeness at hand. But the time I shared with Kevyn went way beyond just physical proximity. He was always more interested in what lay beneath the beautiful mask he was creating on the canvas of your face. He wanted to know what was really going on in there. It takes such courage and honesty to relate to people that way, and as far as I can see, that is how Kevyn approached everyone. He was an intensifier. He laughed louder than anyone and cared more deeply, therefore encouraging you to be that much more in touch with your emotions.

I feel so blessed that my work has brought me close to extraordinary people like Kevyn. Many of the times we shared together were spent shooting with Irving Penn. There is one job that particularly resonates with me as being extra special. We were shooting the couture collections for *Vogue* in this old, abandoned artist's atelier in Paris. Now, from my understanding of the time, Mr. Penn had not shot couture in Paris outside a studio in decades, so the environment was almost holy. We all knew that we were creating something really special.

It took almost a week to shoot everything, but that in itself was a gift, to have the time together to create something we could all honor and appreciate. The moment had such a timeless quality to it. The pictures that resulted were so special, but more important was the experience that I shared with Kevyn. During that week in Paris, our relationship began to transcend the business we were in, and we embarked on an unforgettable friendship. We shared ourselves completely.

When I think of him now, I remember him standing in front of the open windows with a Big Mac in one hand and his *Deep Thoughts* joke book in the other as we listened to *The Little Mermaid* soundtrack. We would laugh at some random *Deep Thought* and in the next moment cry over some line from *The Little Mermaid,* all during the quickest, most stunningly creative makeup changes ever.

I've always admired Kevyn for his commitment to his values and beliefs. I know that some of the same forces he fought against growing up in Louisiana, like racism and homophobia, are what he continued to wage battle with as an adult. He felt compelled to share this mission with anyone who would listen. Some people found it exhausting, yet Kevyn never shied away from speaking out. He felt it was his personal duty.

Kevyn was so generous, but not only in the way that people typically think of generosity. He always managed to remember your birthday with beautiful flowers or a card or a gift, but beyond that he was generous with himself. He brought himself fully to every situation and to every person in his life. That is the gift that Kevyn gave me, that is what he taught me, and that is what still lives on with me.

Shalom Harlow

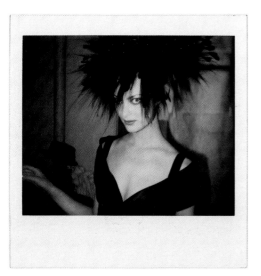
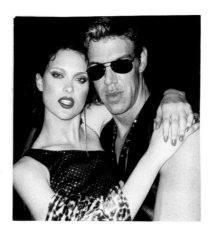
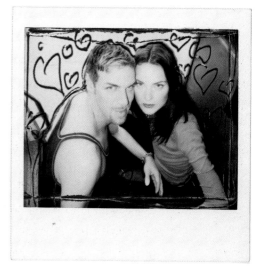
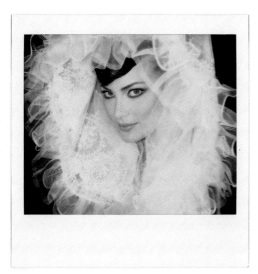
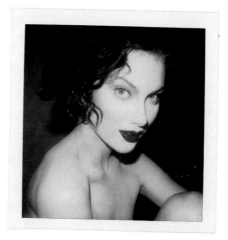
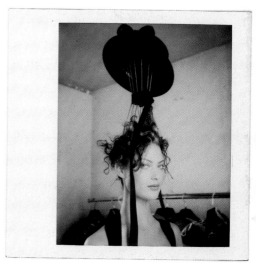
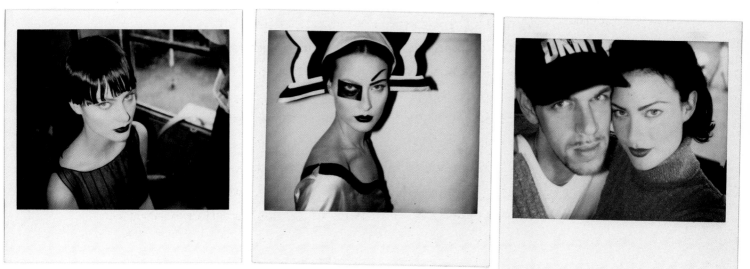

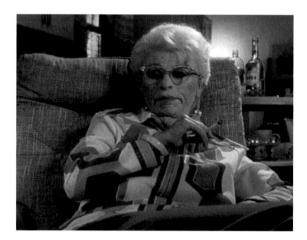

I was made aware of Kevyn by Caroline Rhea when she told me how much he liked my work. Then he mentioned my makeup artist character, Ruby Romaine, in the dedication list of one of his books. We met in New York at a sad event, the memorial service for Liz Tilberis, the late editor of *Harper's Bazaar.* He was so strong and manly and gallant. He and his partner, Jeremy, said they would take Katie Couric and me home, but first we stopped for a drink, and we ended up talking fondly about Liz and having a happy, positive evening.

I thought Kevyn was wonderful, so looking for a laugh, just like me. We started to exchange funny tapes. His staple that he sent to everybody was a Raquel Welch television special from the 1970s with Bob Hope, Tom Jones, and John Wayne. It's unwittingly hilarious. I have since ordered about fifty copies! I also sent him many of the things I find funny, including a great tape I have from a news source of a couple being arrested in Tennessee.

The woman is very indignant, and as she shouts at the police, her dentures fall out on the sidewalk. Kevyn and I talked about this tape for hours, imitating the woman, dissecting every moment of this debacle. "Did you see her husband's Mellow Yellow T-shirt? How about the police car door not shutting because everyone was so heavy it got stuck on the pavement!"

Nobody got it the way he did. We would talk for hours about what made us laugh, real people, and his childhood in Louisiana. It seemed that neither of us had had it easy, with lots of strange relatives, alcohol, and no money.

He only did my makeup once, as Edith Piaf for the *Today* show, and it was a wonderful experience. He came to my apartment to get me ready, but before we started, he had to show me another funny tape. It was of a high school performance. A boy and a girl gyrated to a Rod Stewart number, lots of teased hair, lip gloss, and spandex. The guy

Tracey as Ruby Romaine.

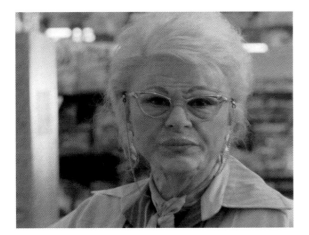
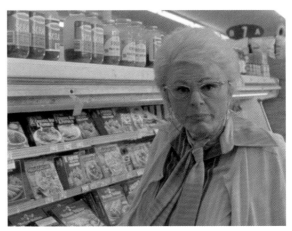

started a series of *Fame*-like split-jumps, ending with an unfortunate landing that caused him to lie injured on the stage. What made us howl was that the other dancers didn't stop. They just danced around the guy and stepped over him when they took a bow. It was very funny to us, but what made me laugh most was watching Kevyn watching it.

When he finally made me up, he told me to lie back on a pillow on the floor. It was so comfortable. I asked him why he did it this way, and he said that was how he made up his sister when they were kids. I have been made up many, many times, transformed by Oscar-winning prosthetic artists. I've seen it all, but that day I was so impressed. He shaped my flat, low-browed, Eastern European face into Piaf's little sparrowlike one. He gave me a heart-shaped face, cheekbones, hollow 1930s eyes. It was incredible. All as I lay back comfortably with him talking and making me laugh. It was such a lovely experience.

I have just finished an HBO show about Ruby, my makeup artist character, and have dedicated it to Kevyn. He loved her. She's a white, union blowhard, alcoholic bigot. She has a son who is damaged from the Vietnam War called Buddy, and her heyday was working on *Bonanza* and powdering Eisenhower's nose for Oval Office addresses. Kevyn loved to talk to me as if I were Ruby and have me insult him. "You're a sissy who's stolen all my ideas, and you don't know what you're doing! I've worked with the best—Hedy Lamarr, Vic Mature, Ruth Buzzi!" He particularly liked the fact that Ruby had her first kid with her uncle, so the child called him "Uncle Daddy."

There aren't that many people who make me laugh, but Kevyn really could. He was a great man, so liberal and curious. I would have loved for him to make up some of my characters. He could have showed me how to cut down on using so much rubber and glue.

Tracey Ullman

I first met Kevyn ten years ago on a cool October night at a restaruant in the West Village. A mutual friend, Robert Montgomery, who was visiting from New Orleans, had told me for years about his good friend Kevyn, whom I had to meet. He thought we would have a lot in common and that we would become fast friends. Little did he realize that our first encounter would lead to the most significant relationship of my life.

As we sat around the small, crowded table in the dimly lit restaurant, I instantly was caught up in what I call the Kevyn spell. The gleam in his eyes, the handsomely unconventional face, the warm, friendly voice, the brutal honesty, and the devastating wit were so appealing. I fell hard for Kevyn . . . and fast. We ended up talking into the wee hours of the morning, and after I left I was walking on clouds. Because of his hectic schedule, I didn't believe that we would see each other so soon. But two days later I got a call from him, and our relationship took off. My life was to completely change. Kevyn would open my mind and my world. He would share with me his love of life, introduce me to everything he was passionate about, and also change my view of the world. He would teach me about self-acceptance. Kevyn would show me that nothing was worth doing if you didn't do it with all your heart. Most important, he taught me about the true meaning of unconditional love.

We spent five and a half years together as a couple. When our relationship ended, Kevyn assured me that his love would not change, only the dynamics of our relationship would. This was a hard concept for me to grasp. But once again, Kevyn would prove to be my greatest teacher in life. When he entered into a new relationship, he continued to include me in every aspect of his life. After all, we were soul mates, he would say. I remained his business partner and oversaw his professional life. We were like family. His devotion to me as a friend never wavered. When I needed him, he was always there. Through his actions, Kevyn showed me that it is possible to love many people in many different ways. Kevyn had the capacity to do so and believed that we all could, if we just opened our hearts to it. I was always amazed to see how Kevyn treated everyone the same, no matter age, race, or sex. All with the same open, loving heart.

When Kevyn passed away, I was at his side. I remember how peaceful he looked. I remember feeling that he had accomplished everything he wanted, even though his life was cut so short. His message, "Seeing the beauty in everyone and everything," is timeless. Now that he is gone, I have made a commitment to carry on his legacy. I know that he would have done the same for me.

Eric Sakas

Photo by Michael Thompson

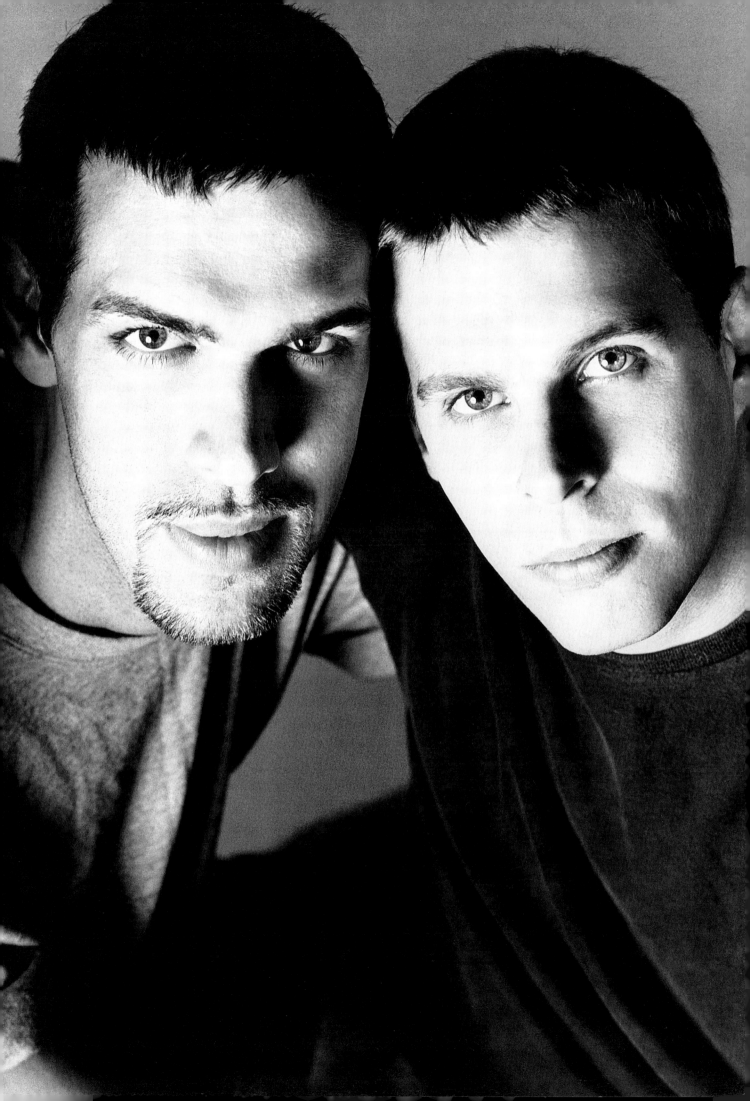

I was planning my wedding back in 1993, fretting over every flower, napkin, and matchbook like any nervous bride. There was no deliberation, though, over whom I would ask to do my makeup. It was my big moment in the spotlight, and, like an actress going to the Oscars or a singer making a music video, I had to have Kevyn Aucoin. If I could get him. Another makeup artist asked me about my plans, and I answered, simply, "Kevyn." She went silent. Then, somewhat ominously, she said, "Don't let him gild the lily."

The rumor going around about Kevyn at the time was that he was—gasp—heavy-handed. Like all rumors, this one was disparaging on one level and comical on another. Kevyn was the undisputed king of makeup. He practically invented the natural look. His rivals had to dig up something, and this was the best they could do. After all, Kevyn could transform a model into a supermodel; an ingenue into a star; his mother, his neighbor, his boyfriend into Marlene Dietrich, Billie Holiday, Linda Evangelista. That kind of hocus-pocus often involved elaborate taping, overdrawn lip liner, and vats of contour cream.

Kevyn put the rumor right in its place. Backstage at a fashion show, while a movie camera filmed the action, Kevyn narrated his technique on

Kate Moss. "I'm not going to give Kate foundation," he said, echoing every makeup artist at the time. "I'm just going to put on a little bit of concealer, just light makeup, only where she needs it." And then he scribbled that fat, fleshy stick all over Moss's nose, cheeks, forehead, and chin until she was as covered as a geisha. They both dissolved in laughter.

Kevyn could gild the lily or, by some combination of sorcery and skill, make that lily look fresh and full and touched only by dew. But skill alone didn't explain why Kevyn was the most admired makeup artist in memory. He had a mission, and he needed everyone to hear and understand it— quickly. His message was: You are beautiful, every single one of you.

The irony was that he proselytized with makeup. In magazines. At fashion shows. Could there be a world more obsessed with surfaces and slickness? Could there be a more unforgiving arena? But Kevyn loved the impossible quest, the lost cause, the dark horse.

Kevyn's passion grew out of his own experience. He spent the first part of his life feeling awkward and ugly and the second part reconciling that feeling in himself. Over and over, in the pages of magazines and books, he explained his philosophy and his methodology so that every woman (and man) would be able to sit in front of a bathroom mirror with a bunch of makeup and follow his lead. He knew that pigment and powder could deliver something far more compelling than fuller lips or thicker eyelashes. It could build confidence. Kevyn had a way of discovering the potential of every person he touched and bringing it to light.

Just the other day, a group of *Allure* readers gathered to talk with me about the magazine. One said, "I miss Kevyn. You should find someone else like him." I was so startled by the pain I felt that I had to stop for a moment and take a breath.

Kevyn and I worked on one of his last columns for *Allure,* a particularly personal essay about being an outcast as a boy in Lafayette, Louisiana, and why beauty became such an overwhelming drive for him. One paragraph was particularly thorny. He called me from a photo shoot, from a car, from an airplane. We revised, bickered, rewrote, debated. On a Saturday morning, satisfied with the piece, he read it to me, his voice trembling. "Today," he read, "I see beauty everywhere I go, in every face I see, in every single soul, and sometimes even in myself."

I miss Kevyn, too. And there's no one else like him.

Linda Wells

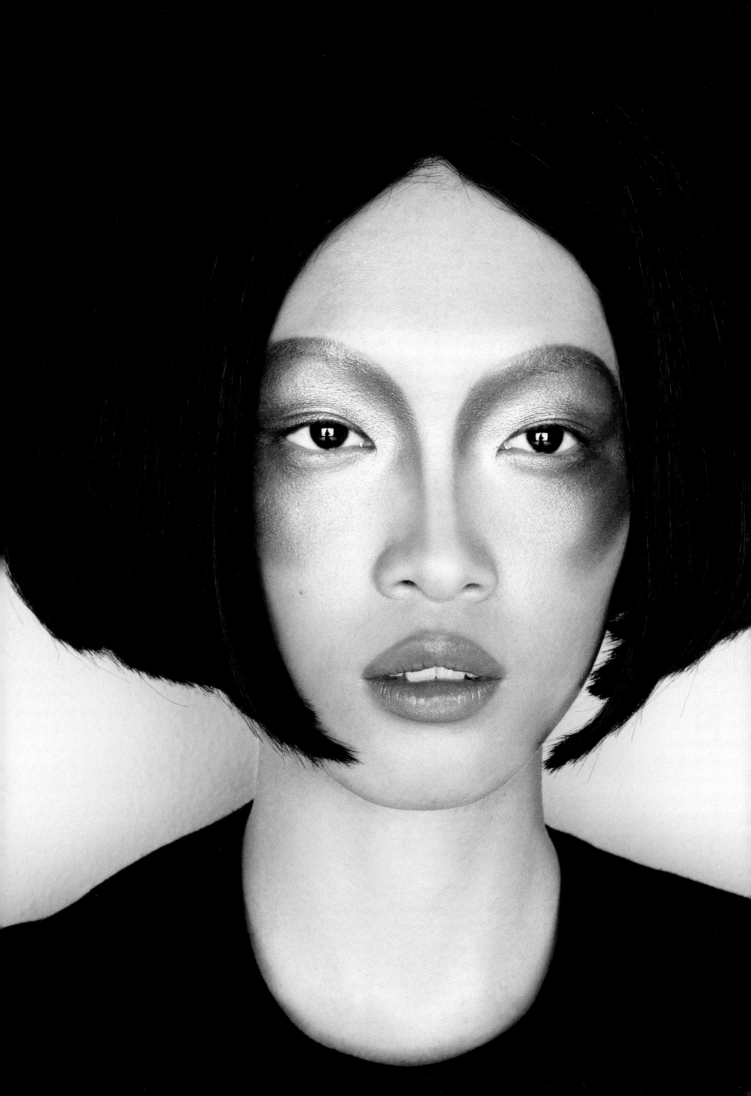

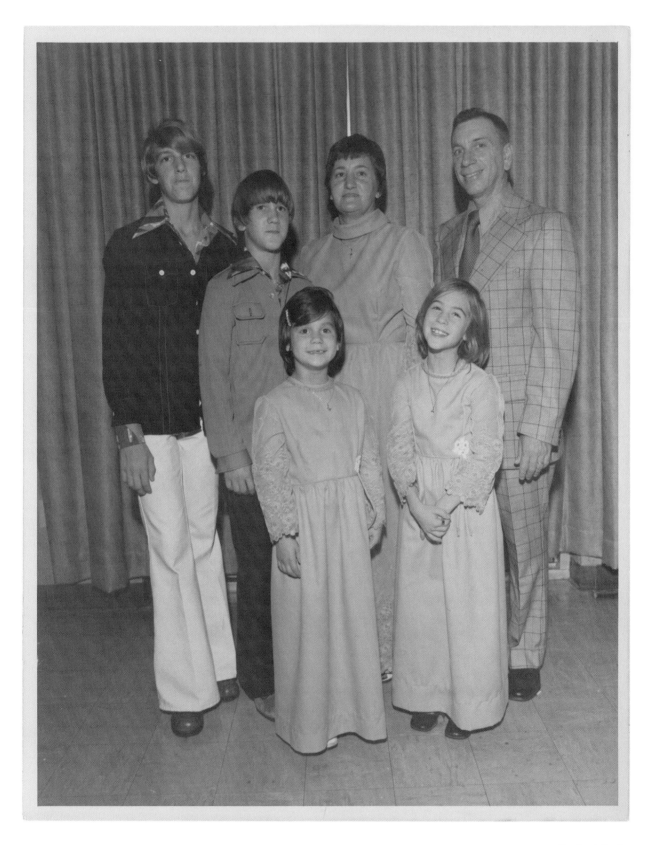

The Aucoin family.

1962–1977

CHAPTER ONE

THE FOUNDATION YEARS

"I understood early that beauty was power."

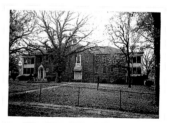

"I MADE A CRASH

LANDING HERE ON EARTH

ON FEBRUARY 14, 1962, IN

THE SHREVEPORT

CATHOLIC CHARITIES HOME

FOR UN-WED MOTHERS. THE

INFAMOUS BONNIE AND CLYDE

LOST THEIR LIVES JUST

MILES FROM WHERE I WAS

BORN. LIKE OUTLAWS OUR-

SELVES, MY BIRTH MOTHER

AND I WERE ON THE RUN

FROM THE DAY SHE FOUND

OUT I WAS PART OF HER."

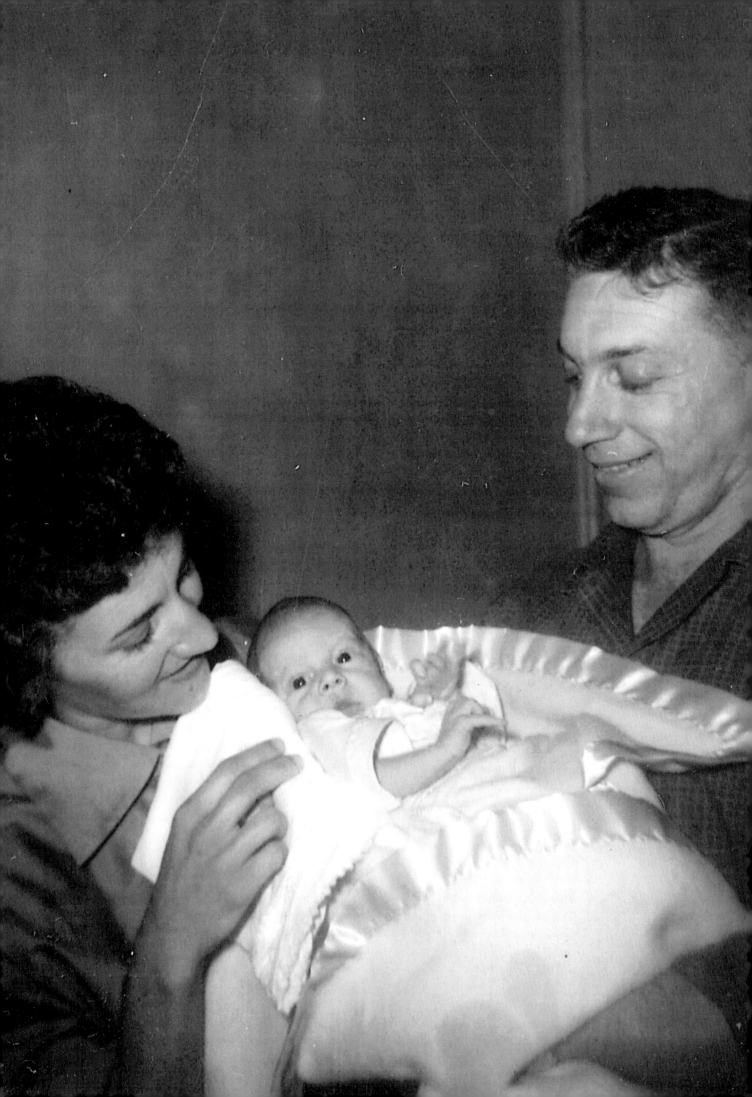

As an adult, Kevyn Aucoin led the kind of glamorous, fast-paced life that can only be imagined. He tended to the face of every A-list star, penned best-selling books, met princesses and presidents, and commanded thousands of dollars for a single day's work. Few could have predicted this incredible rise given his heart-wrenching childhood.

The complications began well before Kevyn was born. His mother, Nelda Mae Sweat, was a scared, pregnant sixteen-year-old with strict Baptist parents. His father, a handsome football player named Jerry Burch, didn't believe that the baby was his. When Nelda's parents discovered her condition, they shipped her off to St. Ann's, a home for unwed mothers in Shreveport, Louisiana, where she lived for three months. Nelda went into labor on Valentine's Day and almost died during the delivery when her blood pressure dropped precipitously. Her parents forbade her to see the baby boy, but she managed to slip into the nursery each night and rock him to sleep. She named him Scott Kevin.

Right before she was discharged, Nelda made one last secret visit to the nursery. She clipped off the baby's ID bracelet and returned home,

heartbroken about the child she was forced to leave behind. She had no idea if she would ever see him again.

Across the state in a town called Lafayette, Isidore Aucoin, Jr., a telephone company manager, and his wife, Thelma, had filed an adoption request with the Catholic Charities and were put on a waiting list. The couple, childless after a decade of marriage, desperately wanted a baby. A month later, while Thelma was washing dishes in their modest home, the phone rang. A newborn was available.

The Aucoins named him Kevin James. (Almost twenty years later, Kevyn would change the spelling of his first name.) Thelma doted on her baby, and he grew into a plump, jowly toddler. "When he was two, he was so fat his legs would rub together until they were raw," recalls his aunt Laura Bourgeois. "The pediatrician made Thelma put him on a diet, and Kevyn cried and cried."

By this time, Kevyn had a baby brother named Keith, who also came from St. Ann's. Over the next eight years, two adopted girls rounded out the family—Carla, gregarious and feminine, and Kim, tomboyish and introspective. The girls shared one

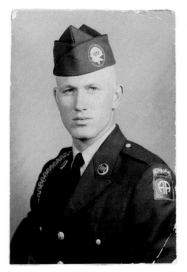

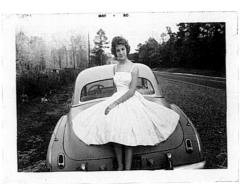

Opposite page: Thelma and Isidore with their new baby.
Far left: Jerry Burch.
Above left: Nelda Mae Williams.

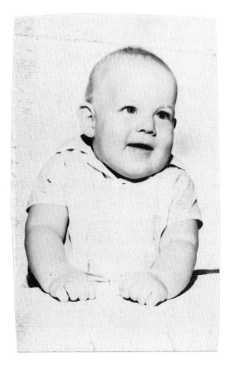

bedroom and the boys another in the red brick house that Isidore had built years earlier in the middle-class neighborhood. The Aucoins had a carport, a big backyard, and one bathroom. The monthly mortgage payment was $74.66.

Like other little boys, Kevyn liked to climb trees and run around barefoot. But he also loved to dance, draw, and listen to songs (such as "Raindrops Keep Falllin' on My Head") over and over. "I was a regular little boy who also enjoyed things that girls did," Kevyn told the producers of *Oliver Button Is a Star,* a documentary based on the 1979 children's book *Oliver Button Is a Sissy.* "I was a tomboy and a sissy boy." Kevyn wore bright green patent-leather loafers on his first day of school and regularly rearranged the living-room furniture—both with his mother's approval. "She was very supportive of me being who I was and understood my femininity," said Kevyn. "That gave me the impetus to be who I am today."

By the age of six, Kevyn realized he was different from the other kids, but, he said, "I didn't know what gay was. There was no such thing when I was growing up. I knew I had crushes on boys, but I didn't think there was anything wrong with that until I started to hear about it from the other kids in school." Even the local Catholic priest ranted about evil homosexuals during his sermon every Sunday. Kevyn thought he was destined to become a rapist or a child molester. He first considered suicide at the age of eight.

He tried to fit in, but it was tough in a town like Lafayette. Located in the heart of Cajun country, it wasn't a progressive or tolerant place by any stretch. At its best, it was a tight-knit society that embodied the joie de vivre of the Cajuns. At its worst, it was a population of small-minded, insular folks, wary of anything or anybody different.

At the age of eleven, Kevyn tried to bury his feelings about boys and found a girlfriend named Karen.

kevyn aucoin: a beautiful life

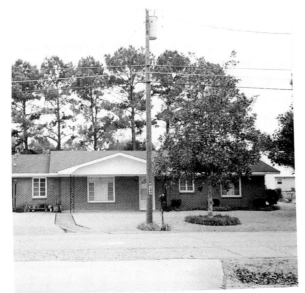

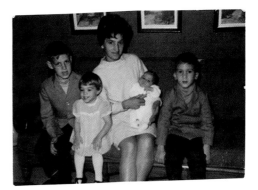

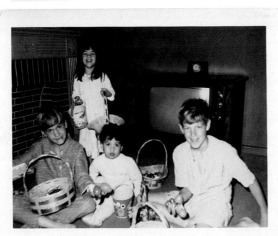

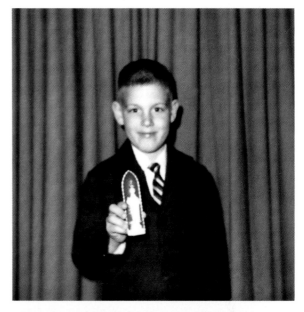

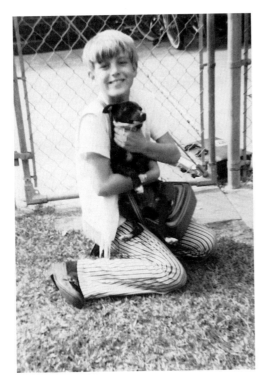

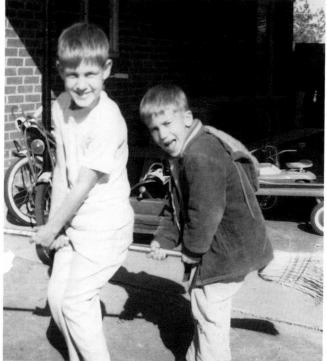

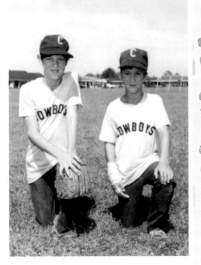

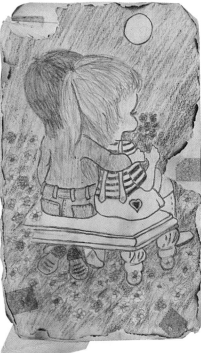

DEAR KEVIN,
THANKS SO MUCH FOR
EVERYTHING YOU GAVE ME
WHILE I WAS DOWN, THE
NECKLACE, THE LITTLE BOOK
AND ALL THE OTHER BOOKS.
I'LL RETURN THEM SOME-
DAY ALONG WITH YOUR
JOHN DENVER ALBUM. WE
MIGHT JUST KEEP YOUR
CARPENTER'S TAPE! (JUST
You made my day! KIDDING)
LOVE,
Karen

They wrote love letters back and forth and talked about getting engaged. "If my family ever moved out of this city, I'd run away and come back to you," wrote Karen on her baby-blue notebook paper.

Kevyn played baseball to please his father, who coached Kevyn's and Keith's teams. He was a Boy Scout, but the crushing separation anxiety he suffered when apart from his family made the required camping trips an impossibility. He was an accomplished saxophonist with the school band until his instrument was stolen. The Aucoins could not afford a new one, so his music career came to a halt.

Gangly, effeminate, and artistic, Kevyn became a target for his classmates. The physical and verbal abuse began around the fifth grade. "We'd be at the bus stop, and they would use words like *faggot* and *queer*," says his brother, Keith, who today is a welder and a father of five. "I didn't know what these words meant, but I knew they hurt him. They would spit on him, slap him across the head, and punch him. I didn't understand what was going on, but Kevyn was crying, and I needed to do something. I'd jump on somebody's back and get my ass beat, and Kevyn got beat, and then we'd walk home." Isidore Aucoin remembers the day Keith tried to rip through a screen door to get at some boys who had been taunting Kevyn.

Many of the teachers in Kevyn's elementary school turned blind eyes to the torture or even participated in it. One male teacher "made a habit of bringing me in front of the class, taking my pants down, and spanking me, which was sexual abuse, basically," Kevyn said. "It's something that I look back on and just cringe. It was a horrible, horrible

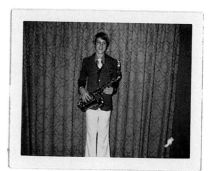

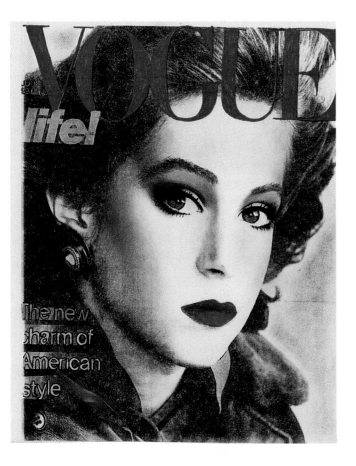

experience." To add to the humiliation, Kevyn often was summoned to a speech therapy class—via a schoolwide intercom announcement—where a young female teacher tried to eradicate his lisp.

Things at home were as stormy as Louisiana's subtropical weather. "Fights with my father were really quite brutal," said Kevyn. "I would not live his vision. I would not become who he wanted me to be. Everything I did was criticized. I would spend three months drawing something and show him, and he would look up from his paper and just look back down. I got no approval from him for anything I did that was creative."

On top of all this, his parents were alcoholics. Looking back, Isidore says he didn't realize how his drinking or his behavior affected his son. "Kevyn seemed to think I was an alcoholic, and I guess I was," he says, sitting at the kitchen table in the family home. "I'm not going to try to deny that. I did

drink, and I drank almost every day. Thelma and I both drank. I didn't go to bars. Nothing like that. But I did drink at home. I don't think it affected my relationship with the kids. I might have thought I was doing all right, and maybe I wasn't."

Despite Thelma's drinking, Kevyn adored her, as she was more understanding of her oldest child than her husband was. "If they had both been unsupportive, I'd be in a mental ward right now—or maybe not even here," Kevyn once said. Thelma's biggest issue regarding his apparent homosexuality was safety, and she thought she could scare him into changing his sexual orientation for his own well-being. Whenever the local newspaper sensationalized a gay-related beating or murder, Thelma clipped it out and left it for Kevyn to see.

Kevyn managed to find several escapes from the turmoil. At the age of eleven, he began making up his little sister Carla, inspired by the glossy

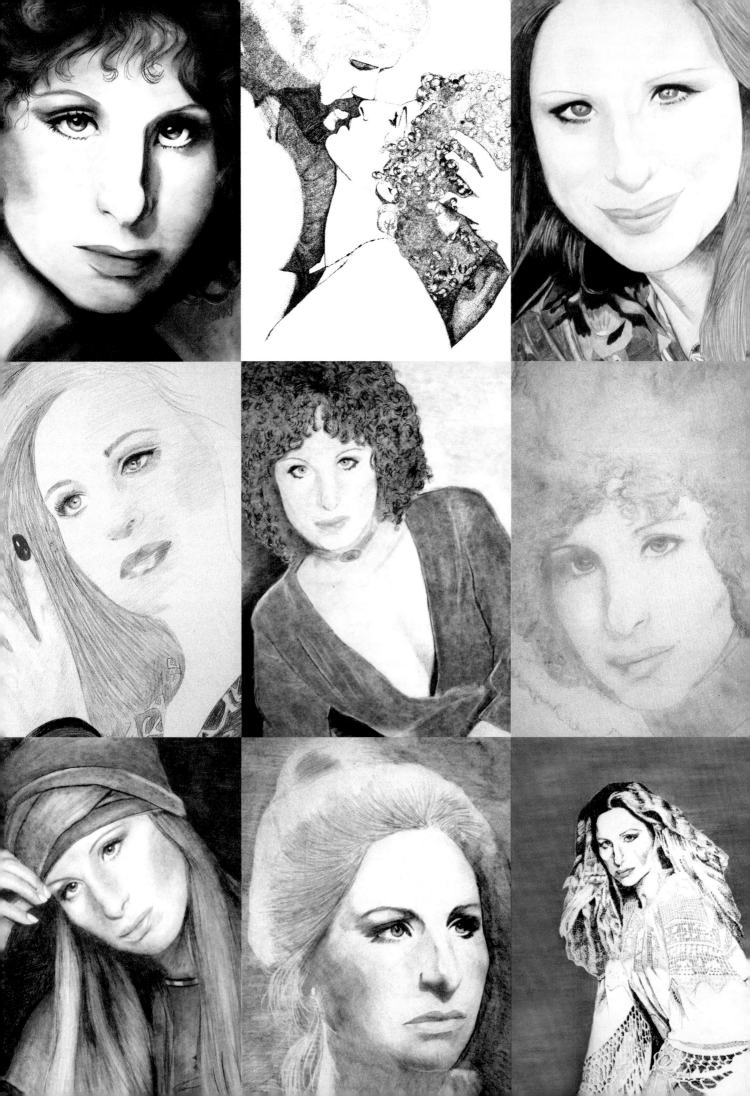

fantasy world featured in his bible, *Vogue.* (Kevyn couldn't afford to buy fashion magazines, so he flipped through them at the local stores, behavior that only added to his reputation as a strange little boy.) He memorized the work of photographer Francesco Scavullo and makeup artist Way Bandy and transformed his barely six-year-old sister into a disco diva, Brooke Shields, or supermodel Rene Russo using a handful of props, some fabric, and a few cosmetics borrowed from Thelma's very limited supply. When Kevyn finished with the hair, makeup, and wardrobe, he tacked a rug or a sheet to the wall, positioned Carla in front of it, and took a Polaroid. The pictures and poses were amazingly mature for two kids at play.

Kevyn's other passion during his adolescence was drawing. "I was absolutely lost in love and life when I did my drawings," he said. "Time stood still." While Carla was his makeup muse, Barbra Streisand was his subject of choice for painting and sketching. Kevyn labored over dozens of portraits of her that he copied from Streisand's movie posters, album covers, and promotional pictures.

By the time his first year of high school rolled around, his obsession with Streisand was full blown. He kept scrapbooks filled with her press clippings, sent her cards on her birthday, and played her music every chance he got. (Isidore remembers hearing "The Way We Were" more than a hundred times.) He owned every album she released, even though he could barely afford them. "Records were expensive," says Keith, who preferred Led Zeppelin and AC/DC to his brother's beloved songbird. "We had to wash the car and mow the grass, rake everything, and then hustle some money around picking up cans and turning in bottles to get things like that."

Kevyn was an outsider among his fellow students, but he never hid what made him different. "There was absolutely no mistaking in most people's minds that he was gay," says Glenn Neely, Kevyn's first serious boyfriend. "That did not go over well." This didn't stop Kevyn from convincing the editors of the Lafayette High School newspaper, the *Parlez-Vous,* to write a story about his Streisand fanaticism. The four photographs that

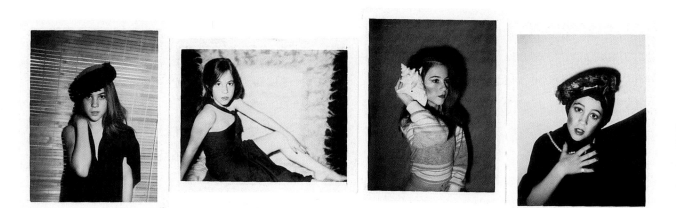

Opposite: Kevyn's drawings of Barbra Streisand. Above: Carla, with makeup, hair, styling, and photography by Kevyn.

accompanied the article were taken on Kevyn's side of his wood-paneled bedroom, which was a shrine to Barbra. "Because of Kevyn's great interest and respect for Streisand, he has started a small but growing fan club," wrote student Lisa Farnsworth in the story. "After graduation he plans to go to California for his senior trip in order to meet her. (Let's wish him luck!)"

The article caught the attention of Glenn, a handsome, blond senior from a well-off family. "I opened the paper, and there was a picture of Kevyn and all the pictures of Barbra all over his wall. He just seemed intriguing to me, and he looked really cute, so I wanted to meet him. I don't know why. I just knew there was something about him."

Glenn, who says he didn't realize he was gay at the time, was on the lookout for Kevyn that day, but he failed to find him. A few weeks later, while Glenn was hanging out at his girlfriend's house, the doorbell rang. It was Kevyn. Unbeknownst to Glenn, Kevyn and his girlfriend had become pals.

"So he walks in, and I'm freaking," says Glenn. "He sits down and starts talking to us and he was really funny, even back then. Within like fifteen, twenty minutes, we decided to walk outside and sit on my car. We left my girlfriend inside. We had a tape deck, and we played music and talked for an hour. We hit it off right away."

Glenn called Kevyn soon after that night and asked for his help finding a tuxedo for the prom. Summer vacation rolled around, and they saw each other almost every day for the entire break. "I don't think we left each other's side for more than a few hours at a time," Glenn says.

For weeks, it was just an intense friendship. Glenn stayed over at the Aucoins', or Kevyn stayed at Glenn's, which was across town in a wealthy part of Lafayette. One late night at the Neelys', the relationship moved to a new level. "I woke up because Kevyn's arm had fallen over on me. I sort of froze. I didn't know if I should do anything or pretend it wasn't there," says Glenn. "Eventually I put my arm around him. Within a few days, we moved upstairs and started sleeping in the same bed."

Around this time, Kevyn officially came out to his mother. Thelma had been raised Catholic and was taught that homosexuality was wrong, but she loved her son and handled his announcement the best she could. "It took us a long time to accept, not just tolerate, but really accept Kevyn being gay," she wrote years later. Thelma eventually left the Catholic church.

The first person Kevyn ever came out to was his cousin, Jay Theall, who was also gay and lived across the state in Lake Charles. Jay was a frequent and intense pen pal who struggled with his emotions and looked to Kevyn for support and reassurance. On the lighter side, they bonded over their fascination with celebrity. Jay's letters in those pre-e-mail days were filled with references to movies, award shows, Top 40 countdowns, and a whole cast of '70s stars, led by their absolute favorite, Barbra Streisand. "Did you see the American Music Awards? Linda Ronstadt beat Streisand! I wanted to be sick. I couldn't believe it," wrote Jay in one of the dozens of letters Kevyn saved from his cousin.

With the summer coming to a close and school a few weeks away, sixteen-year-old Kevyn thought

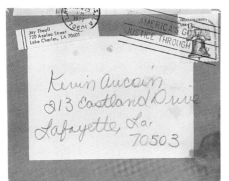

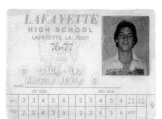

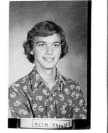

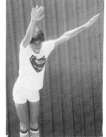

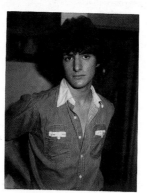

Kevin Aucoin
213 Castland Drive
Lafayette, La.
70503

Jay Theall
720 Azalea Street
Lake Charles, LA 70601

AMERICA'S GOAL: JUSTICE THROUGH LAW

ACADEMY AWARD WINNER BEST SONG "The Way We Were"

3-22-77

Hello Kevin,
Listen, I have a few minutes and I just thought I would tell you on April 24, 1977, Barbra Streisand is going to have her 35th Birthday! This is what I plan on sending her— It's a charm on a chain

(Over)

35 Congratulated women

Barbra 1977

Do you think it's a good idea, write back and tell me!

Bye,
Jay

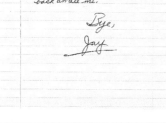

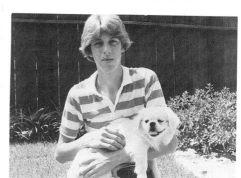

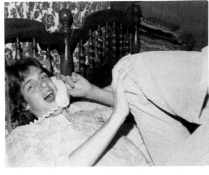

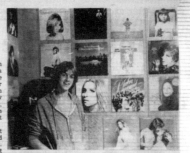

Reflections of Our Time!

Beauty is in the Eyes of the Beholder

By LISA FARNSWORTH

Kevin Aucoin, a sophomore at Lafayette High School, has a hobby that many of us would find rather unusual. He is one of the biggest fans of Barbra Streisand.

Kevin has collected T-shirts, twenty-seven of her albums, four posters, and seven scrap books from her childhood to present. He has seen A Star Is Born six times, What's Up Doc? five times, On A Clear Day You Can See Forever four times, For Pete's Sake three times, Hello Dolio, Funny Girl, The Owl and the Pussycat, and The Way We Were. Using a special camera, film, and recorder he has taken pictures of and taped A Star Is Born, What's Up Doc&, and For Pete's Sake.

Kevin has delved into the life and career of Barbra and found she was born in Brooklyn, New York in 1942. She grew up knowing lonliness and death, for she grew up without her father. During her childhood and high school days, her fellow students called her Crazy Barbra and Big Beak. She then started living up to their conceptions of her. She went to the movies as an escape from her lonely world. After Barbra left the theatre, she would return to her home to stand in front of the mirror and re-enact the character she had previous seen. Upon her

graduation from Eramus High School with a 4.0 average, Barbra began working at a Chinese Restaurant to earn money for Malden Bridge Playhouse, an acting school in Malden, New York. In the Spring of 1961, Barbra launched her career in singing at the Lion, a restaurant on Ninth St. in Manhattan.

Kevin has written letters, sent her a birthday card, and received pictures signed by her in return. Because of Kevin's great interest and respect for Barbra, he has started a small but growing fan club.

After graduation he plans to go to California for his senior trip in order to meet her. (Let's wish him luck!)

When asked for a personal opinion he commented, "Barbra is the only person ever to receive every entertainment award, a feat which she accomplished before the age of twenty-five. She is not a teeny bopper fad! If you are a fan of hers, you appreciate her work in all aspects, singing, acting, and composing music. Barbra stands her ground, is original and can never be duplicated."

Obviously, Kevin strongly identifies with Miss Streisand because of similarity in their backgrounds and physical characteristics.

Kevin Aucoin, a fan of Barbra Streisand.

Feelings confusing
stirring longing
from deep within
a sense of
security
for living
attempting
striving
to be me.

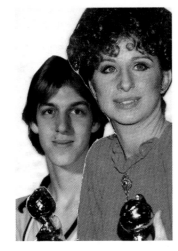

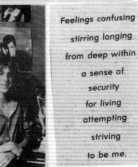

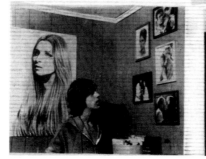

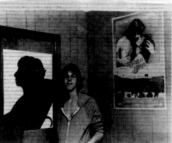

Below: Kevyn and Glenn, in and out of costume. Opposite: Diana Ross drawing by Kevyn.

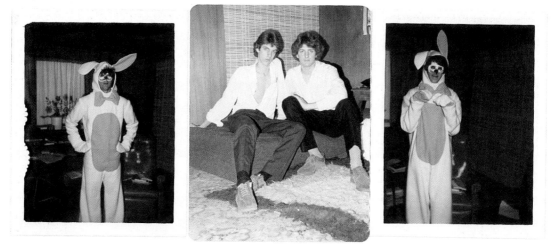

he and Glenn should live on their own. Neither of them had a job, and their only money was a $250 benefit check that Glenn received each month because his father had died in a plane crash when he was a baby. All they could afford was a dingy one-bedroom apartment a few miles away from the Aucoins' that rented for $200. They had little money left over each month, so they relied on their parents for food and other basics.

Flush with their newfound independence, they decided to visit their first gay bar, a local joint called Southern Comfort. "We had heard these horror stories about gay bars and that it was this big orgy, so we were petrified to go in," says Glenn. The two waited outside for what seemed like hours, but the street out front wasn't a safe place to be. Every now and then, some locals drove by and threw bottles at the entrance. "It wasn't a bad part of town—it was just a bad thing to be gay," notes Glenn.

It was the height of the disco era, so when the two finally worked up the courage to run inside, they found a dance party under way. Donna Summer's big hit "MacArthur Park" was on the sound system, and Kevyn and Glenn were surprised to see men dancing together.

Later that night, they met their first drag queen: Ms. Pool. These men made up as women mesmerized Kevyn. It was a pivotal moment, as he was witnessing firsthand the transforming power of makeup. If you wanted to be someone or something else, all it took was the right products. You could literally change your life—or someone else's—with lipstick. After his encounter with Ms. Pool, Kevyn started inviting drag queens over to his apartment to do their makeup. Soon enough, all of them wanted this sixteen-year-old prodigy to paint their faces.

That September, reality beckoned. Kevyn had to start his junior year of high school and Glenn his freshman year at the local college. The taunting and abuse that began in grammar school had yet to end for Kevyn. "From the day I started high school, I was beaten up daily," he said. "I spent every recess hiding in an empty storage room." Kevyn finally dropped out after some students tried to run him over with a pickup truck. "I quit because my life was threatened, literally."

A month later, Glenn dropped out of college. As he was no longer a student, this meant the end of his government checks. The two teenagers now were broke, but they were in love and on their own for the first time in their lives.

In 1994, Kevyn would tell *The Advocate* that meeting Glenn had saved his life.

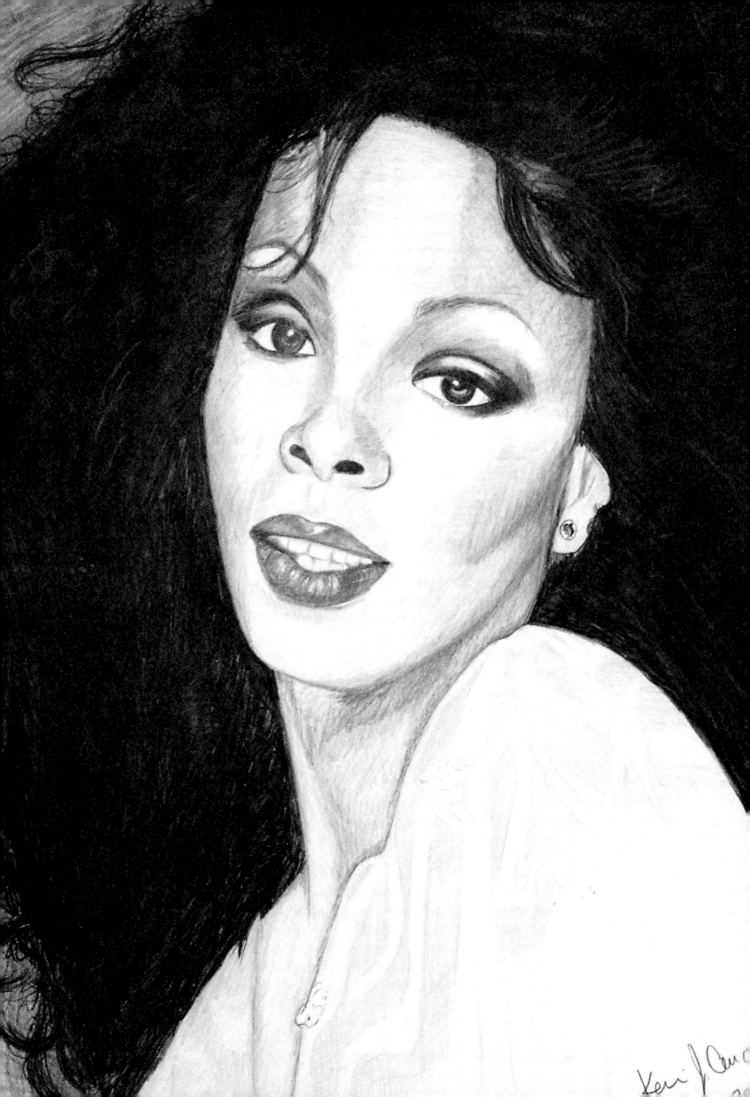

"I was like Pluto. I was so outside the norm. And I was okay with it."

CHAPTER TWO

THE INDEPENDENT YEARS
1978–1981

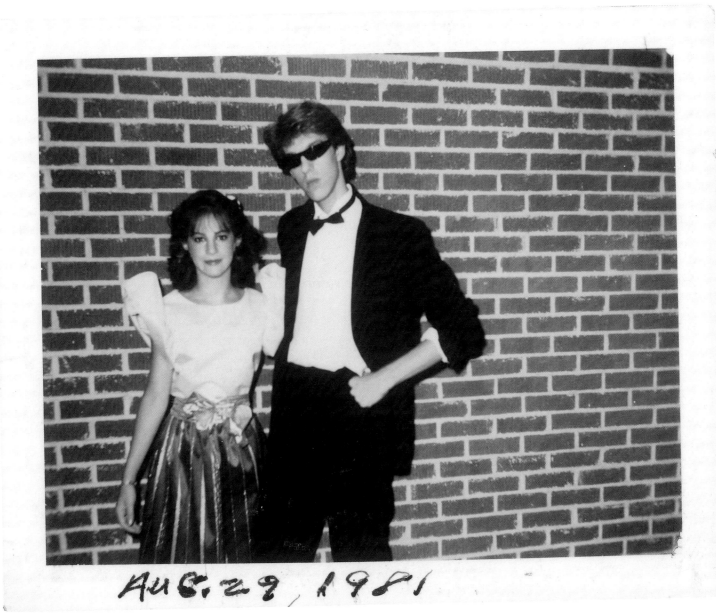

AUG. 28, 1981

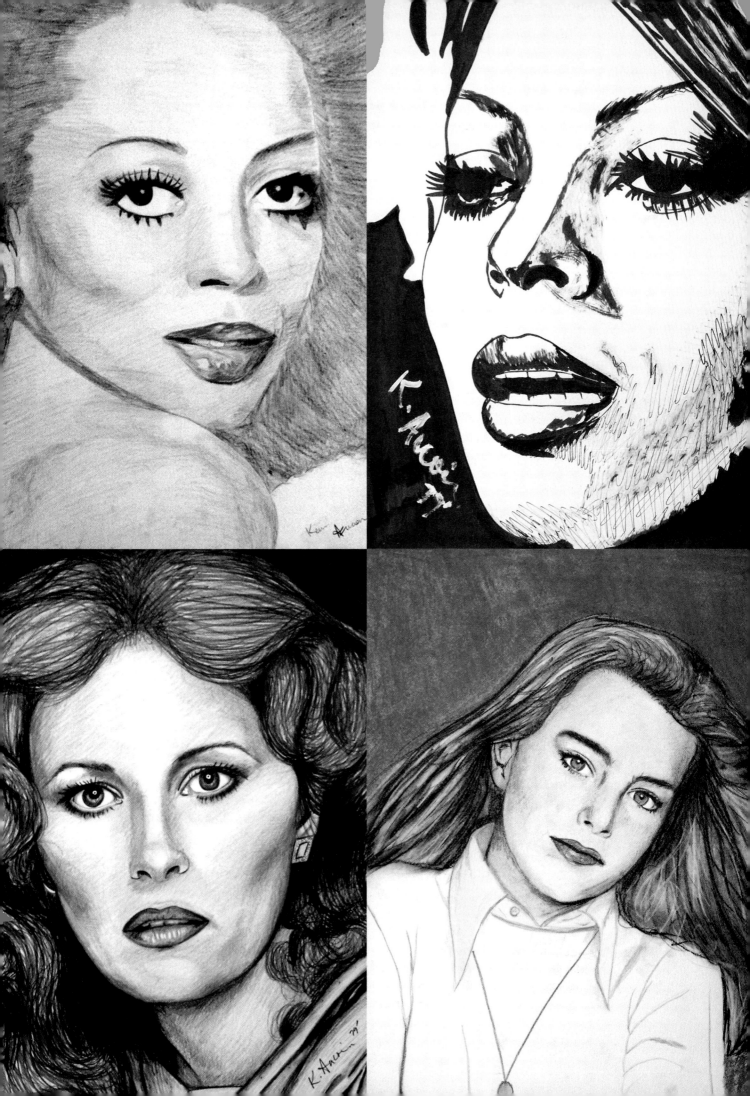

Kevyn and Glenn had no money to pay the rent, buy groceries, or go out, so somebody had to get a job. And that somebody was Glenn, who found work, of all places, at the phone company with Kevyn's father. The unlikely pair commuted together every day.

Kevyn and Glenn moved several times in their three years as a couple. Their second apartment was a room above a garage in a bad part of town. Kevyn stayed home all day and would draw, update his Barbra Streisand scrapbooks, pore over his massive collection of fashion magazines, and do makeup on Carla, Kim, his drag-queen friends, even Glenn. They shared their next apartment with "two gay guys, a twenty-five-year-old virgin, and a prostitute," according to Glenn. "Kevyn once caught her shaving a lightning bolt in her pubic hair," he laughs. "We thought that was the weirdest thing we'd ever heard of in our entire lives."

Because Kevyn had no money, everything he owned—his records, magazines, and makeup— had been shoplifted. "He would go to the store and take a sack with him and just put tons of stuff inside it and walk right out the door," says Glenn. "I was with him when he got caught, and that was the last time he ever stole anything."

Sometime after he dropped out, Kevyn decided to give school a second try. It was a place where he thought he would definitely fit in: beauty school. He asked his father for $900 to cover the tuition. "I said to him, 'I can take this goddamned money and dump it in the sewer,' " Isidore recalls. "I just didn't see him making a living like that."

Isidore eventually handed over the cash. Deep down, he wanted Kevyn to succeed, and besides, his son could be extremely persuasive. "When he had a goal in his head, he'd go over you, under you, or right through you to achieve it," says Kevyn's sister Carla.

Beauty school was a waste of time and money, but not for the reasons Isidore envisioned. Most of the curriculum centered on hair, and Kevyn knew more than the teachers when it came to makeup *and* hair combined. "I hoped they would show me secrets and help me to become a 'professional' makeup artist," Kevyn said in later years. "Little did I know that in between hiding in the laundry room so I wouldn't have to do anyone's hair, the teacher for the makeup class would be me!"

Kevyn eventually found a job in the cosmetics department of a local store. It didn't last long because some customers were offended by the idea

kevyn aucoin: a beautiful life

51

of a male makeup artist. Kevyn's next job was at the most posh boutique in town, Sandy Austin Ltd. in the Acadiana Mall. She sold the best designers around, such as Bill Blass, Calvin Klein, and Geoffrey Beene, and chic beauty brands like Erno Laszlo and Madeleine Mono. This was the closest Kevyn had ever gotten to the names he read about in his favorite fashion magazines. "He loved that job," says Glenn. "He started making a living at doing makeup, which was a whole new concept to him."

Sandy Austin, a single mom with three children and expensive taste, had opened the store when Lafayette was in the midst of an oil boom. Before then, local women had to fly to New York, Houston, and Dallas to spend their nouveau riches because there was nothing to buy in town. "There was more money being made here than you can imagine," says Sandy.

One of her seamstresses happened to be Thelma Aucoin. "She had these holy pictures over her sewing machine, and she would be praying novenas, and she'd say, 'I'm praying for Kevyn. Oh, Kevyn's gonna quit school, or Kevyn's gonna do this and that.' One day, she said, 'Would you consider hiring Kevyn, because he *loooves* to fool with makeup?' And so I did."

Kevyn felt his name wasn't unique enough for his glamorous new job, so he decided to tweak it slightly. Inspired by Barbra Streisand, who had dropped the second *a* in her first name, he changed the spelling of *Kevin* and replaced *Aucoin* with the name given to him by his birth mother. He was now, as Sandy Austin billed him in an advertisement, "Kevyn Scott, makeup artist and skin specialist."

Kevyn proved to be an enthusiastic addition to Sandy's staff. "He was a very gifted employee, but just . . . hyper. I mean, if Kevyn took two steps back, he knocked something over and broke it. It was like having a colt in a china closet. He liked to sleep late, so he would come in at twelve and work

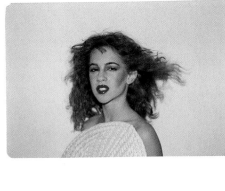
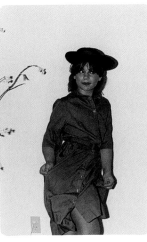
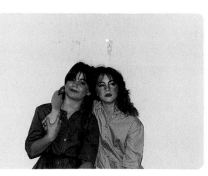

Above: Sister act—Carla and Kim.
Opposite: The Aucoin siblings by Kevyn.

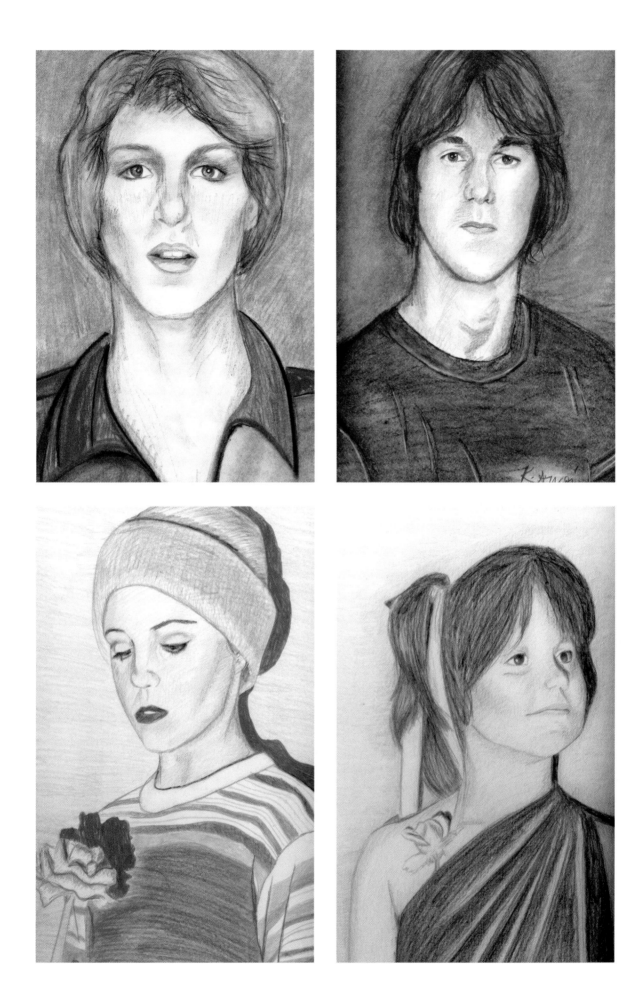

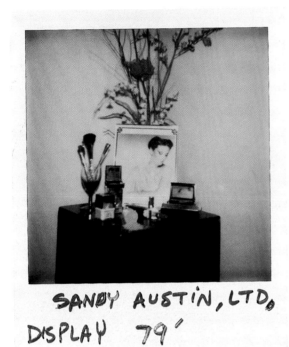

SANDY AUSTIN, LTD.
DISPLAY 79'

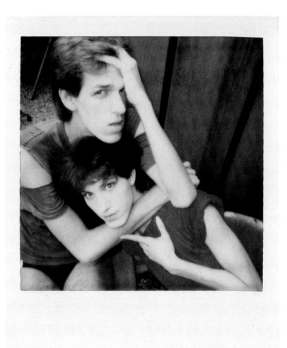

until eight P.M. If business was slow, he would snag somebody and get in the window of the mall and draw a crowd doing makeup. People would come in the next day and say, 'I was in the mall last night, and Kevyn was doing a little show in the window!' "

Kevyn had never been on a plane and had never left the South until he accompanied Sandy on a business trip to California. "He brought a holy picture with a novena on it that Thelma had given him," says Sandy. "He was so nervous he prayed all the way to L.A.!" Several months later, she took him on a buying trip to New York and brought him to the designers' offices. It was a short visit, but he fell in love with the city. He thought each New Yorker who walked past him was a celebrity. "I said,

'Kevyn, everybody in New York is not a star!' and he said, 'Well, I think they are!' "

Although Sandy adored her young employee, she fired him—twice. "He became unruly, and I didn't have the time to control him. I'm sure Kevyn had ADD [attention deficit disorder], but in those days, it wasn't a buzzword. He would entertain all the salespeople at night, and they wouldn't do what they were supposed to do. Or he'd get in the window and do makeup. I'd have corrective interviews with him and say, 'Kevyn, you can't do that. If you're not busy, take inventory of your cosmetics so we can reorder. Don't play around.' "

Another issue was Kevyn's flamboyant friends, who used the boutique as a hangout. "One of them had green hair, and they all wore black," says Sandy. "They were just . . . different. And, you know, we're talking the '80s here, before all of this came on the scene. I said, 'Kevyn, you know this is a high-end store. This is not gonna work.' "

One of those friends was Scottie Vaccaro, who had moved from Baton Rouge to Lafayette and met Kevyn through a friend of a friend. Scottie introduced him to New Wave music, such as Holly and the Italians, the B-52's, XTC, and Ultravox, which they'd bring to local bars and ask the DJs to play so they could dance. "We were like cool outcasts,"

what I felt, and that's not what I thought of myself as, so they used to give me trouble." But not Kevyn. "He was very happy about it because he could do my makeup."

Kevyn always painted Scottie's face before a night out. "We're talking fifty pounds of makeup. Kevyn wore makeup, too, maybe something on his mouth, some eyeliner, mascara, a little blush on the cheeks. We'd get all made up, and we'd have all this hair and these wild clothes, and we'd just go out and tear it down." But sometimes the bouncers wouldn't let Scottie through the door.

Sandy Austin
LIMITED

Kevyn Scott
Make-up Designer & Skin Specialist

Sandy Austin LTD.
Acadiana Mall

Welcomes to her staff

Kevyn Scott

MAKE-UP ARTIST & SKIN SPECIALIST

Make-Up Lesson	30.00
Eye Make-Up Lesson	20.00
In Residence Make-Up Lesson	60.00

FOR APPOINTMENT CALL 981-1906

says Scottie, who now lives in New Orleans. "We'd be all punked out."

Kevyn and Scottie bonded over their outsider status. "Growing up, I wanted to be a girl, but I had people saying, 'Little boys don't wear dresses. Little boys don't do this. Little boys don't do that,' " remembers Scottie. "I didn't realize that I wasn't a little girl until all this started clicking in. After that, I just shut down. I would spend all my time in my room drawing and listening to Patti Smith."

Scottie had no confidants because few people, of any sexual orientation, understood the situation. "The gay boys just want you to be some kind of drag queen," Scottie complains during an interview in her French Quarter apartment. "That's not

"They knew I was a boy, but I was dressed like a girl, or whatever. So one night Kevyn wrote something nasty in blackberry-colored lipstick from Revlon on the wall outside. That was Kevyn. I was very low-key, like, 'Kevyn, don't do that.' But Kevyn was, like, 'Fuck them.' "

The shift from frightened underdog to the confrontational Kevyn was under way. Over time, he'd grow confident enough to stand his ground and speak his mind instead of scrawling some graffiti and running away. "As he got older and more successful, he wasn't afraid to say what he thought," explains Glenn. "He thought he finally had earned the right to give his opinion. He was becoming secure in a way that he never was before."

But this growing assertiveness was starting to affect Kevyn's relationship with his boyfriend. "He was always pushing to do what he wanted," says Glenn. "I didn't feel like I had my own life. He wanted to spend hours and hours and hours doing pictures and making up people. His passion for makeup and his dreams for moving up the ladder in the fashion industry were all-consuming."

The two broke up, and Kevyn decided to move to New York. "He said he had nowhere else to go," says Glenn, who eventually headed to California and became a financial consultant and author. Sandy Austin arranged for Kevyn to stay with a friend of hers from Louisiana named Lois Hesterly, whose teenage daughters danced with the New York City Ballet.

Theatrical and motherly, Lois had a twelve-room apartment on 118 West 79th Street, across from the American Museum of Natural History. It was known as the Ballerina Farm, because so many young dancers roomed there. Lois worked as a costume designer during the day and would come home in time to cook big dinners of crawfish étouffée, jambalaya, and other Cajun specialties for anyone who walked through the door. Each night, photographers, dancers, choreographers, musicians, conductors, and theater people would gather around Lois's table to drink, dine, and gossip.

Kevyn had dreamed of a world like this, but it was the right place, wrong time. "He was the sweetest thing, but he was so homesick," recalls Lois's daughter, Melinda Roy, who is now a Broadway choreographer. Kevyn and Lindy, as she was called, would sit around listening to Rickie Lee Jones records on her stereo, and Kevyn, still heartbroken about Glenn and missing his family, would sob along to each song.

To cheer him up, Lindy would drag him to her favorite haunts, Studio 54 and Xenon. "They would attack my wardrobe and find outrageous coats to wear to the clubs, even though they were far too young to be in those places," says Lois. Kevyn and Lindy never had trouble getting in. All the doormen knew Lindy ("because I used to dance my brains out"), and they'd wave the two teens past the velvet ropes.

Kevyn rarely worked, according to Lois and Lindy. Neither of them even remembers him having a portfolio. But Kevyn was confident enough in his talent to arrive on the doorstep of Francesco Scavullo looking for a job. At the time, Scavullo, along with Richard Avedon, ruled the world of fashion photography, and his studio was the center of all that Kevyn desired.

Kevyn had no idea that his idol, Way Bandy, was working with Scavullo that day. "Francesco was

Opposite: Kevyn's copy of Way Bandy's beauty book, borrowed from the library and never returned, and Way's autograph.

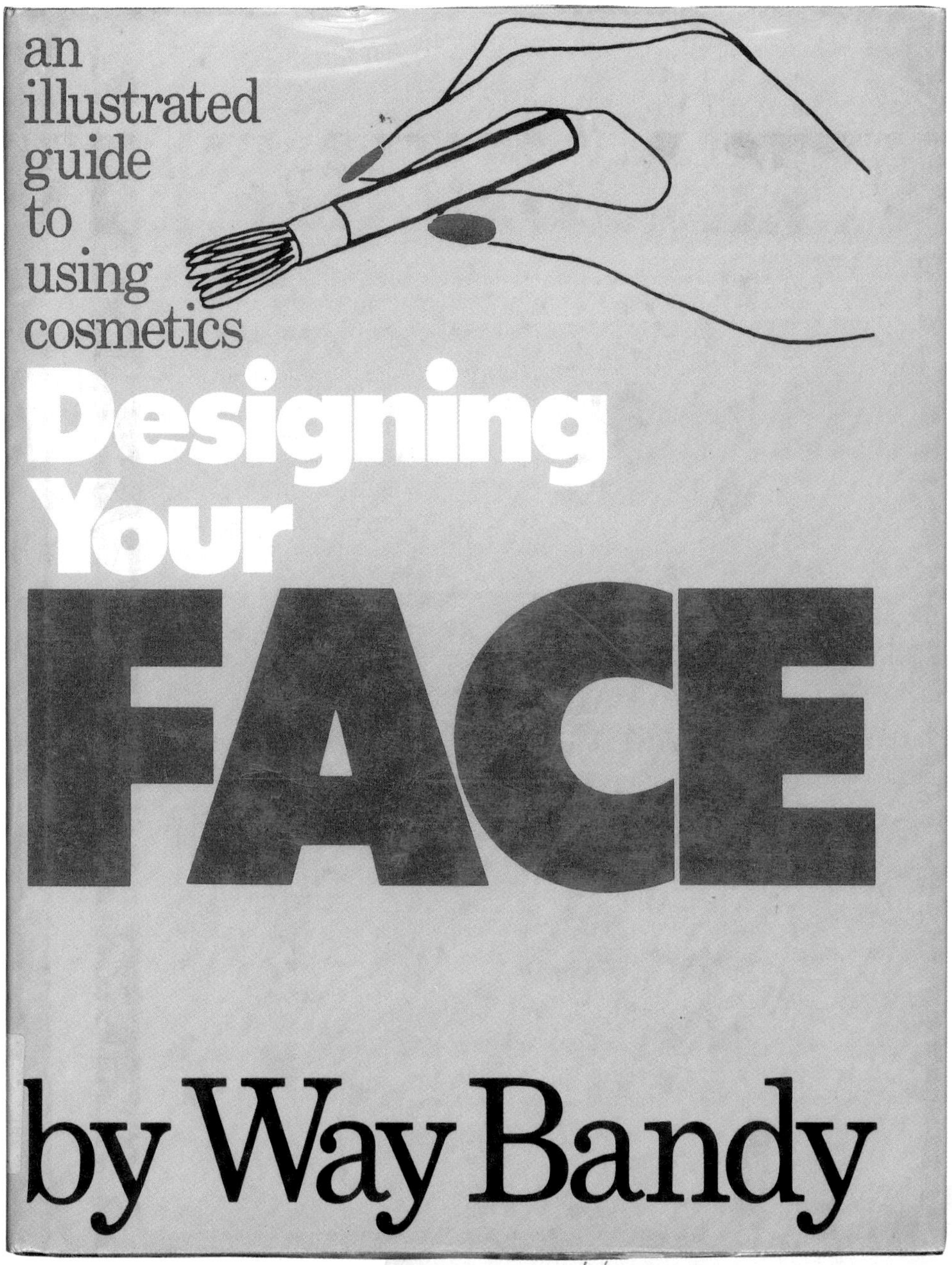

an
illustrated
guide
to
using
cosmetics

Designing Your FACE

by Way Bandy

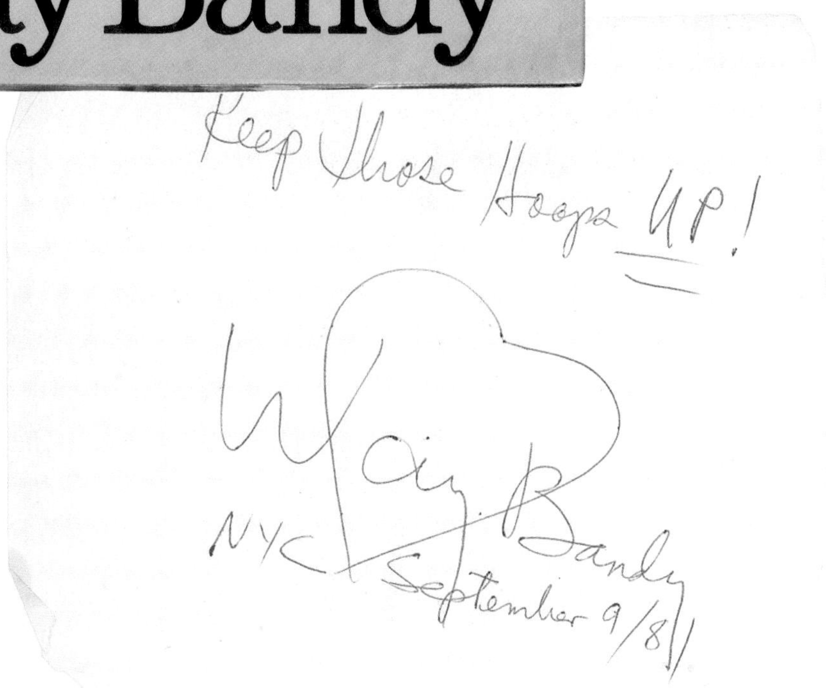

Keep those Hoops UP!

Way Bandy

NYC September 9/8/1

57

Page 1

"NEW YORK"

● Dear Everyone,
Hi, How's Lafayette?
Fine, I hope! How's
school girls? Good!
I hope! ☀ (It better Be!)
I hope Keith finds some
work that he enjoys! Keith, you need
to sit down + write a list of your
favorite things to do + see if their
is work in any of those fields. Check
out all of the possibilities!! Quit getting
jobs that are easy to get, boring to
● do + then end up quitting. Think
about what you want (Set a high
goal or you'll never have to reach up
to get anything + will cease to grow.
+ when you cease to grow, you
die!) + then do it! Kim, Hi! I
hope you're liking school better
this year. Have you made new
friends? I'm sure you have! I'm
constantly looking for things for all
of y'all so keep things in mind that
you might want + write + tell me!
Hi Carla, How is school + life?
● I wish you'd start taking your
vitamins!! "TRY!" Its for your own
good. I hope daddy is taking his!!
(over)

●

I talked to Odelia + she said that
she would be very interested in having
me in her salon! I would lease a
space. I was thinking that when I
came home, you + I could think of
doing something on our own. I
think that would be alot of fun! Maybe
y'all could enclose the back carport!
+ that could be our workroom, my
design room + bedroom. Maybe. Just
trying to think of all the possibilities,
● or Maybe Mathew + I's things will
come through (our store Portfolio.)
who knows? Well I'm glad things
are going well back home. Its freezing
up here! You better hurry + send
me some scarves. Its COLD!
I'm going to do makeup on
all of the people who work at Fiorucci
+ they are going to take a picture of
me + them. Call Kim - 981-8767 and
Roland W. - 981-3155 (He works at the Shoe Str.
in the Acadiana Mall) go + tell him I said
"Hi!" Well better say "Bye" See y'all
● soon! I love y'all! write me!
L♥VE,
KEVIN

58

FORD MODELS, INC.
344 East 59th St., New York, New York 10022
(212) 688-8538
Telex 234443 - F M A U R

To Whom It May Concern:

We at the Ford Model Agency, highly recommend Kevin Aucoin as a superb makeup artist and hairdresser. He has worked with Ford for several months and has unfortunately decided to return home to pursue his craft in Louisiana.

He will sorely be missed and we hope that he will return with his expertise to New York City.

Sincerely,

Claudia Black

Claudia Black
Director of
Ford Classic Women

CB:lmg

shooting the cover for *Vogue* on Karen Graham [who, at the time, was the face of Estée Lauder], so Way was in the dressing room doing her makeup," recalls Sean Byrnes, Scavullo's partner and longtime stylist. "Kevyn comes in, and he has a book no bigger than eight by ten. There were only a few pictures of his family in it, but I looked at it and said, 'Oh, I have to show this to somebody.' I'm telling you, it was incredible. So I went into the dressing room and showed it to Way. He comes out and pushes Kevyn on the chest and says, 'Kid, you're gonna go places,' and went back to finish Karen's makeup."

It was a huge moment for Kevyn, as he had learned everything he knew by studying and copying Bandy's work. Back in Lafayette, Kevyn had pored over every page of Bandy's 1977 book, *Designing Your Face: An Illustrated Guide to Using Cosmetics,* until he had memorized all the chapters, including "Eyebrows," "Contouring," and "Artificial Eyelashes." Kevyn had borrowed it from the local library and still had it in his possession at the time of his death.

Kevyn's second encounter with Bandy came when he was walking down Columbus Avenue with Lindy's sister Leslie. In an *Allure* magazine article, Kevyn recalled getting Bandy's autograph: "My teeth were chattering, and I was stumbling over my words. . . . He said, 'Oh, darling, where are you from?' When I told him I was from Louisiana, he said, 'Still in hoop skirts, huh?' So he wrote, 'Keep those hoops up. Love Way.'"

Despite his brush with beauty royalty, Kevyn was ready to leave New York. In a letter to his family, sent in a Ford Models agency envelope with the logo scratched out, Kevyn talked about coming home and leasing space in a salon or opening a store that he would call Portfolio. He suggested that "maybe y'all could enclose the back carport" and turn it into a "workroom, design room, and bedroom" for him when he returned.

Shortly after he mailed the letter, Kevyn packed his bags and flew to Lafayette. In later years, Kevyn would tell the press about almost every aspect of his life, but he would leave out the story of his brief, failed move to New York.

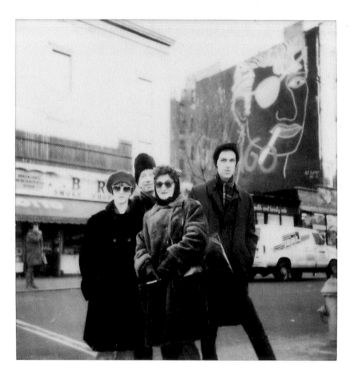

ST. MARK'S PLACE

"Like everyone else, I'm a work in progress."

CHAPTER THREE

THE LEAN YEARS
1982–1985

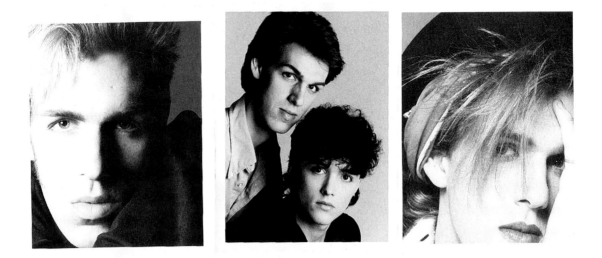

Preceding spread: Carla, Isidore, and Thelma visit New York. Above: Kevyn and Jed Root. Opposite: Scenes from New York.

Despite Studio 54, Scavullo, and everything else New York had to offer, nineteen-year-old Kevyn hadn't been ready for life in the big city. The breakup with his boyfriend and the separation from his family were too much to bear, and he couldn't summon up the drive and determination needed to survive as a freelance makeup artist. Kevyn was happy to be back in Lafayette, but he made it clear to his friend Scottie that his return home was temporary.

In the meantime, he found a job at the Lancôme counter of D. H. Holmes, a local department store. He was a talented salesperson, moving $15,000 worth of products in one month alone, but he and his manager didn't see eye to eye. He soon quit.

One night in February, at a bar in Baton Rouge, Kevyn struck up a conversation with Jed Root, a premed punk rocker at Louisiana State University. They returned to Lafayette together, where they hung out for days, celebrated Kevyn's birthday, and got matching white streaks in their hair. Kevyn was completely smitten. "He is so beautiful! He is so angelic!" he gushed in his diary.

The new couple even bumped into Glenn during Lafayette's Mardi Gras celebration. Kevyn wrote in

his diary that Glenn wanted to get back together with him: "I said no. It was what I have been wanting for eight months. I do love him. But now there's Jed." Less than a month after they had met, Kevyn and his new boyfriend moved into a two-story home on Geranium Street in Baton Rouge. Kevyn called it a "dream house." "Things are going to be great," he predicted in his diary. "I am finally happy."

Baton Rouge wasn't very different from Lafayette in terms of tolerance. One afternoon, Kevyn, Scottie, and their friend Dana were playing with makeup in the beauty department of a local store. Suddenly, a security guard approached the trio and ordered them upstairs. When Kevyn hesitated, the guard reached for his gun. He even banged Scottie's head into a wall before frisking her. The three were threatened with arrest, photographed, and never told what they had done wrong. But Kevyn knew what the problem was: a gay man and his edgy friends fooling around with cosmetics just wasn't acceptable. He discussed the incident with a lawyer but was told he didn't have a case.

Kevyn was quite aware of what it meant to be young and gay—not just in the South but all across

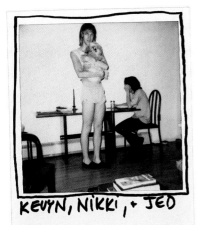

KEVYN, NIKKI, + JED

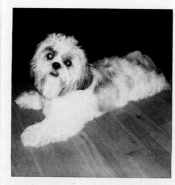

Nikki in N.Y.C.
NOV. (84)

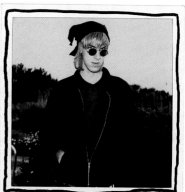

KEVYN IN THE HAMPTONS
AT ARTHER ELGORTS HOUSE

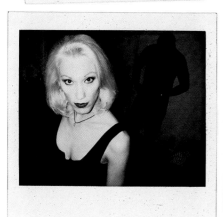

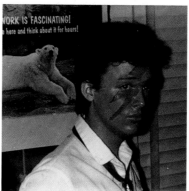

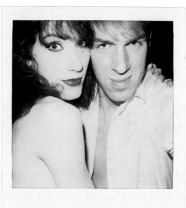

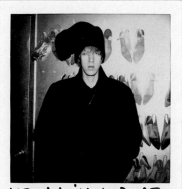

KEVYN IN AND AT
STEPHEN SPROUSE NOV. 84

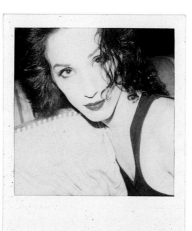

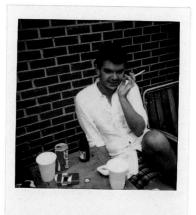

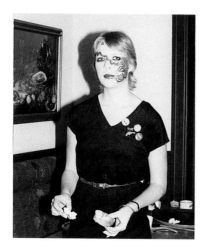

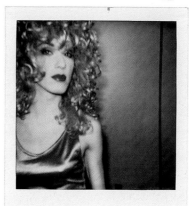

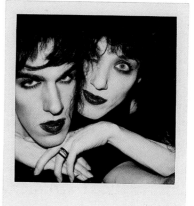

DEBI MASSEY

om first runner-up in a Valdosta, Georgia,
auty pageant to the pages of French Vogue
d L'Officiel, Debi Massey has devoted herself
nodeling with characteristic hard work and
usiasm. And now the soft-spoken 20-year-
ants to do everything—make every cover,
r in TV spots, land an exclusive makeup
t.

'9½" and 120 pounds, Debi has the
nd the bone structure to carry off the
ion clothes that she loves to model—
all gowns or futuristic jumpsuits. To
t those looks, she experiments with
makeup. "It's not just a face," she
reation!"

cial beauty begins with skin care.
r face often, uses cleansing cream
ap, and avoids too much sun. To
damaging effects of hot rollers
she conditions her hair twice a
it a hot-oil treatment once a
s in shape with skating, swim-
istance running, and watches
ause even a few pounds can

e technical basics of model-
onths. However, her work
has taught her the other
er experience grows and
s learning the business of
t lesson for an ambitious
ood mind as well as a

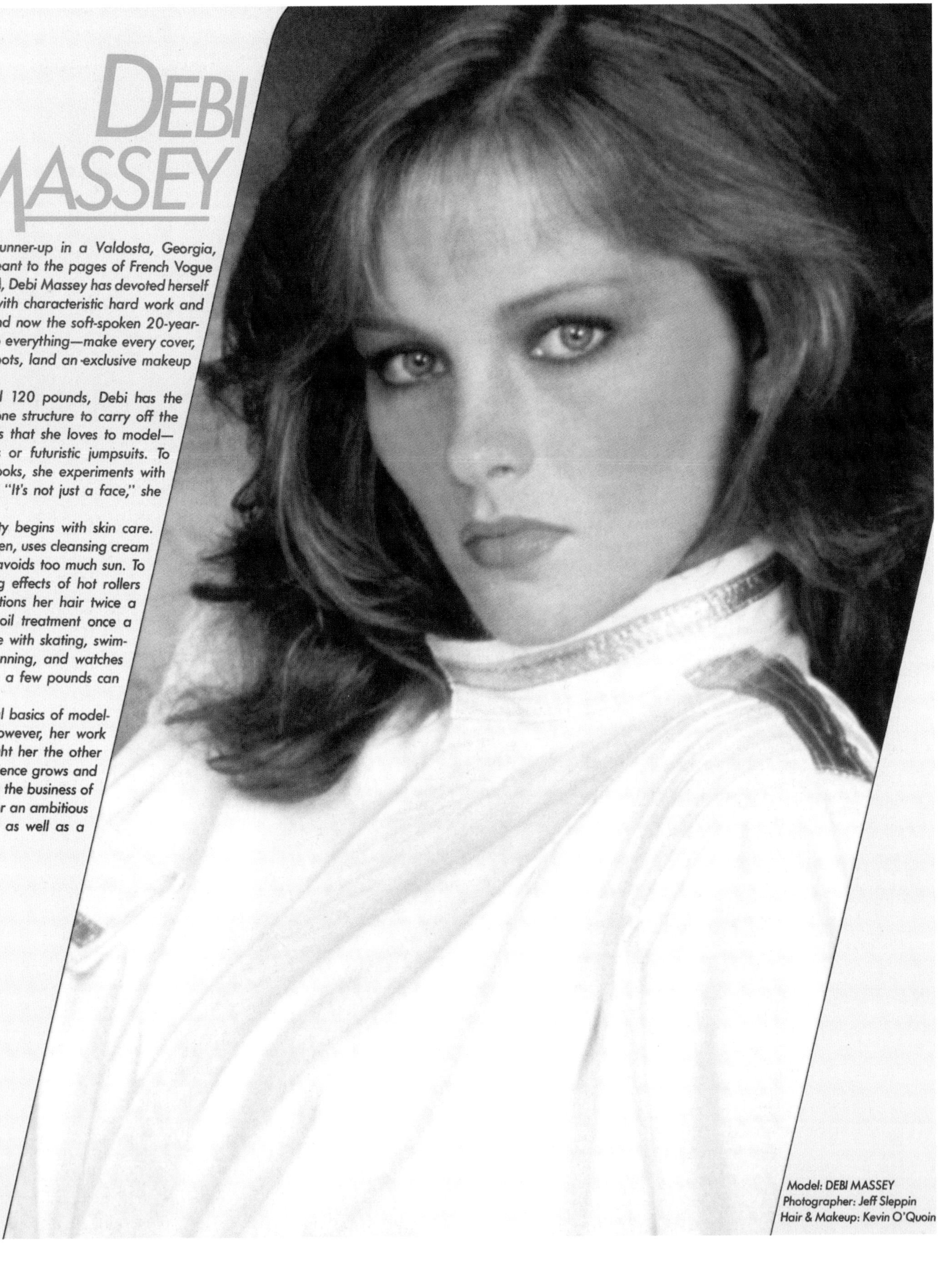

Model: DEBI MASSEY
Photographer: Jeff Sleppin
Hair & Makeup: Kevin O'Quoin

America. At the time, in 1982, Ronald Reagan was president, and Jerry Falwell's right-wing Moral Majority was growing in popularity. The group's homophobic stance prompted Kevyn to send a letter to the *Daily Reveille,* the Louisiana State University student newspaper. In it, he denounced Falwell's followers, explained that homosexuality was not an illness, and pointed out that he was in a healthy, committed relationship with another man. "Our love is stronger than any prejudice or hatred," he wrote.

Shortly after the letter appeared, Kevyn and Jed decided it was time to leave Louisiana. It wasn't the result of any backlash. Rather, Kevyn had walked into a local store and spotted a Ford Models calendar. He flipped through it and was shocked to discover that he had done the makeup for one of the women in the photos. This was the sign he had been waiting for. Within days, he and Jed had packed their

bags. "It was time for him to go," says his brother, Keith. "Down here, he was going to be nothing."

They sold Jed's Volkswagen to the Aucoins for $1,500 and flew to New York, where they moved in with a friend of a friend named Sheila. "She had one of those nasty little tenements with the bathtub in the kitchen," recalls Jed. "The toilet would constantly freeze over." The apartment was on Seventh Street in the East Village. Years later, the neighborhood would be celebrated in the musical *Rent,* and tourists would flock to its bars and boutiques, but in the early '80s, it was a seedy place. "The city was just coming out of its horrible bankruptcy period," explains Jed. "The subways were covered in graffiti, and they weren't safe, so we always took the bus. People told you to hide your jewelry when you walked down the street."

Two months after their arrival, in the middle of a blizzard, and on Kevyn's twenty-first birthday, no

Left: This picture from the Ford Models calendar was Kevyn's first published work. Note the spelling of Kevyn's name in the bottom right-hand corner.
Below: Kevyn's self-portrait and drawing of Jed, featuring their secret language.

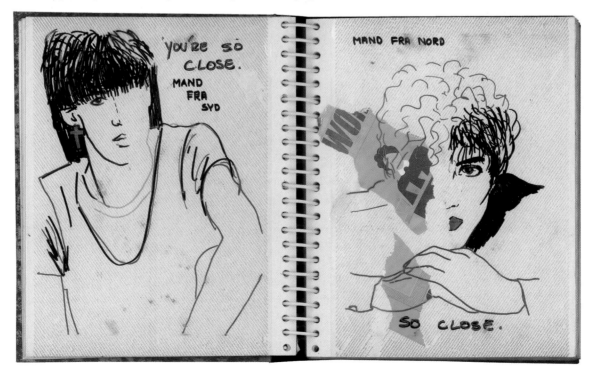

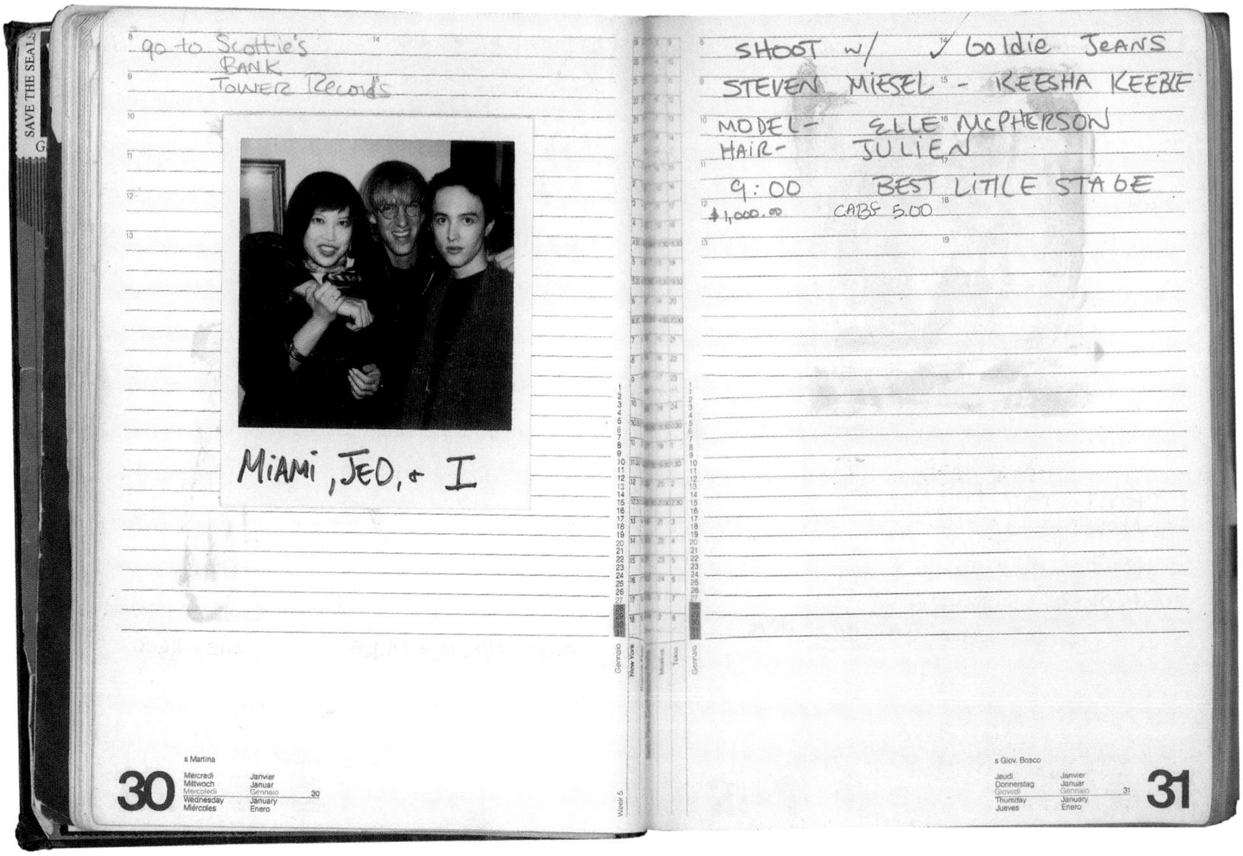

go to Scottie's
Bank
Tower Records

MIAMI, JEO, & I

SHOOT w/ ✓ Goldie Jeans
STEVEN MIESEL - KEESHA KEEBLE
MODEL- ELLE McPHERSON
HAIR- JULIEN
9:00 BEST LITTLE STAGE
$1,000.00 CABS 5.00

30	Mercredi Mittwoch Mercoledi Wednesday Miércoles	Janvier Januar Gennaio January Enero	30

| | Jeudi
Donnerstag
Giovedi
Thursday
Jueves | Janvier
Januar
Gennaio
January
Enero | 31 | 31 |

s Giov. Bosco

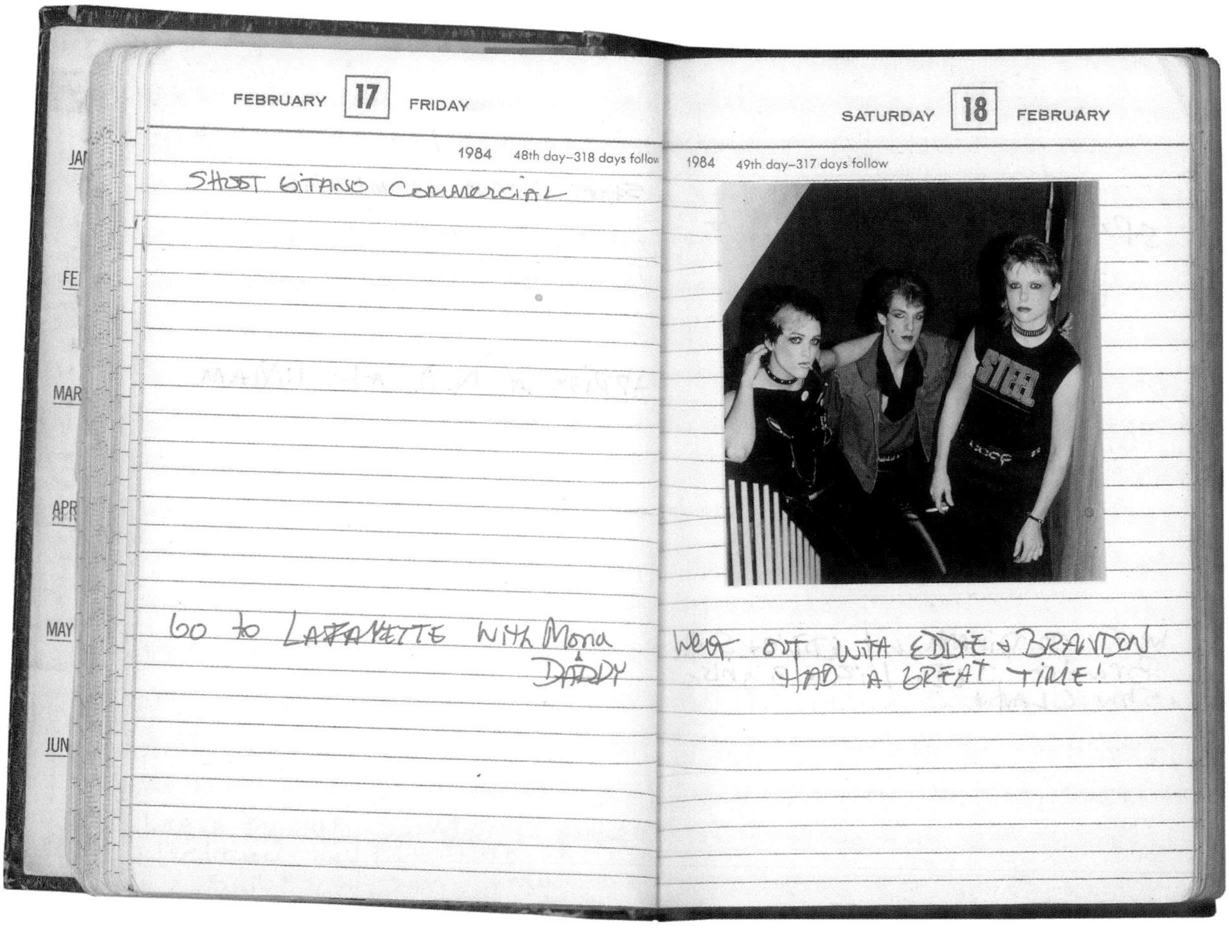

FEBRUARY [17] FRIDAY

1984   48th day–318 days follow

SHOOT GITANO COMMERCIAL

GO TO LAFAYETTE WITH Mona
& DADDY

SATURDAY [18] FEBRUARY

1984   49th day–317 days follow

WENT OUT WITH EDDIE & BRANDON
HAD A GREAT TIME!

less, Sheila kicked them out. They found an apartment at 450 West 46th Street, in a tough part of town known as Hell's Kitchen. "I was starving, got mugged and tested day and night for ten months," said Kevyn. "The apartment was awful. The floor was so old and rotted we couldn't walk on it without shoes, and everything was slanted to the left. We had to get our furniture out of trash bins off the street." Kevyn's sisters came to visit later that year and were less than impressed with the living arrangements. "All you heard 24/7 were ambu-

now and then. Ford eventually paired Kevyn with Lorraine Sylvestre, a French-Canadian photographer who specialized in test shots, which are pictures taken of aspiring models to see what they can do in front of the camera. Kevyn was happy for the work; even though it paid nothing, he got photos for his portfolio in exchange.

His creativity soon caught the eye of the legendary Eileen Ford, but for the wrong reasons. The modeling agency owner told Sylvestre that she wanted these new girls in simple makeup, not the

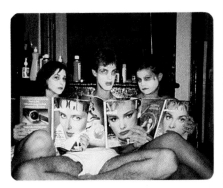 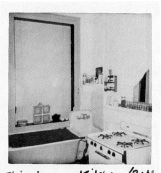 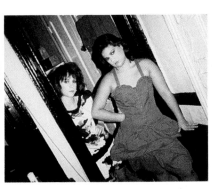

This is our Kitchen/Bath 450 W. 46th 5/27/83

Opposite: Kevyn's datebooks. Above: Carla and Kim on their first visit to N.Y.C.

lances, fire trucks, horns, cussin', and yelling," says Carla. "It was so loud I couldn't believe it."

Still, they showed the girls a good time and took them everywhere, from the Metropolitan Museum of Art to the Circle Line. But for the most part, Kevyn and Jed were broke and existing on a steady diet of ramen noodles. Kevyn was so skinny he said he resembled Meryl Streep in *Sophie's Choice.* Their only friends, some employees at Ford Models, took pity on the duo and treated them to expense-account lunches every

dramatic, contoured looks that Kevyn favored. Lorraine knew it was only a minor bump for the talented young makeup artist. "I sensed he would move on to bigger things," she says. "There was a vibration about him."

Until that big day came, Kevyn needed to make some money. He found work doing makeup for a porn magazine called *Cherry.* The editor in chief, Cherry Bomb, happened to be the most frequently featured model. Soon enough, however, legitimate jobs started to come his way. On one of these, a catalog shoot, he met an up-and-coming Czechoslovakian model named Paulina Porizkova. "He was this little country boy," says Porizkova, who was only eighteen herself. "I didn't expect much when he started. I thought I'd have to sneak into the bathroom and fix my makeup, but I was, like, 'Wow! This guy is good.' "

Kevyn had much bigger aspirations than basic catalog work. He dropped his portfolio at major magazines, but nothing materialized until a photographer named Rob Stern put him in touch with Miami Wong, an assistant at *Vogue.* Miami liked Kevyn's portfolio enough to show it to her boss, *Vogue* beauty editor Andrea Robinson. "Kevyn had maybe eight pictures in his book, but you could see there was real talent there," says Andrea, who today is the president of Ralph Lauren's fragrance business. "I wanted to see more work and meet the makeup artist, so who shows up but Jed, pretending to be Kevyn's agent."

Kevyn's big break came only two weeks later. Makeup artist Alberto Fava had gotten sick very suddenly and couldn't make a *Vogue* shoot with photographer Steven Meisel and a young actress named Meg Tilly, who was promoting her first big movie, *The Big Chill.* "I said to Miami, 'Get Kevyn on the phone,' " recalls Andrea. "To tell you the truth, it was so last-minute I don't think we could get anybody else."

When Kevyn arrived on the set, he told Andrea how excited he was and quickly got to work. "He really had a magic touch," she says. "You could see that right away. He did this soft, very innocent, naive-looking makeup. The eyes were just beautiful." Andrea was thrilled with his work, and so was Meisel. "They clicked immediately, and Steven really helped develop him," says Andrea. "After that

shoot, Steven booked him over and over, and so did I." In less than a year, Kevyn had gone from anonymous, penniless makeup artist to *Vogue* contributor. At just twenty-one years old, his wildest dream had come true. "I think I nearly passed out," said Kevyn in later years. "I remember crying for two days."

Kevyn called home constantly to update his family on his progress. "The phone bill was enormous because he would call collect," says Isidore. "He and Mrs. Aucoin would talk for hours. I'd say, 'What in the hell are you talking about?' He just loved his mother. Let me tell you, he was a momma's boy."

Vogue booked Kevyn again just a week after the Meg Tilly shoot for an assignment with photographer Pamela Hanson and two of the reigning models of the day, Bonnie Berman and Kim Williams. At the same time, Meisel's agency, Art & Commerce, approached Kevyn about representing him, ending Jed's budding career as an agent. "I really didn't know what I was doing anyway," admits Jed, who soon found a job at Name Models. Despite the early setback, Jed would go on to become one of the biggest agents in New York, representing top photographers, makeup artists, and hairdressers.

During the next year, 1984, Kevyn worked for more magazines and with several important photographers—including Peter Lindbergh, Robert Mapplethorpe, Mario Testino, Duane Michels, and Bert Stern. He and Jed found an apartment in SoHo, New York's hot new neighborhood, and bought a shih tzu puppy right before their second anniversary. They named him Nikki, after Porizkova's Russian boyfriend. Kevyn had lots of familiar faces around him. Both Dana and Scottie had moved to New York, and his best friend,

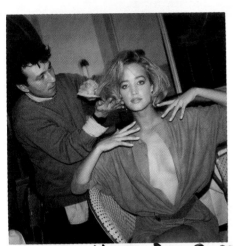

VOGUE SHOOT. Dec. 9 83'
PHOTOGRAPHER - Pamela HANSON
Howard Fugler & BONNIE BERMAN

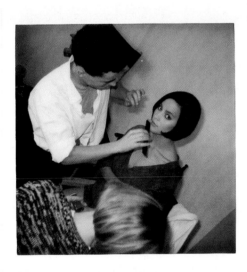

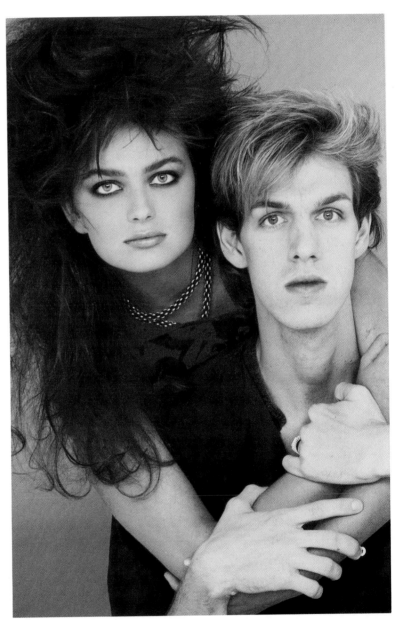

Clockwise from top left: Bonnie Berman, Kevyn with Paulina Porizkova, and Meg Tilly.

ISSUE NO. 432 · OCTOBER 11TH, 1984 · $1.50 U.K. £1.20

Rolling Stone

TINA TURNER
She's Got Legs!

FRANKIE GOES TO HOLLYWOOD
England's Music Sensation

TOM WOLFE
'The Vanities'

STYLE
Rebel without a Cause, 1984

Eddie Greene, visited frequently from Louisiana. Their hangouts included a dive bar called Nightbirds, the famous nightclub Danceteria, and Kevyn and Jed's apartment, where they would do makeup, take pictures, and make funny videos for hours on end.

Kevyn, meanwhile, became the "unofficial mascot" of the *Vogue* beauty department. "He hung out with all of the assistants, telling us stories, making us laugh," recalls Linda Wells, the future *Allure* editor in chief who was an editorial assistant at *Vogue* back then. "He seemed to be there all the time."

Kevyn had worked with a few minor celebrities at this point, but in August, he painted his most famous face yet, Tina Turner. It was for a *Rolling Stone* cover with Meisel that would become one of the most iconic pictures of Tina ever taken. Yet it represented a milestone to Kevyn for different reasons. "I wanted to put these silvery lips on her that

since I was young," he said. "Oddly enough, this was a great relief. The illusion that so many of us grow up with—that something outside ourselves will heal us—was just that: an illusion. Now came the hard part. I had to fix myself—arrgh. I flung myself into therapy with the same passion I had for makeup."

Tina Turner would prove to be part of the healing process. Over the next fifteen years, the two would work together on countless photo shoots, public appearances, videos, and concerts. Through it all, Turner taught Kevyn about spirituality and became, as he described her, his second mother. "I think Kevyn had respect for the life that I have lived," says Turner. "We talked intimately. He talked about his past a lot, and I would give him other ways to look at things. We had therapy sessions, so to speak. I always tried to encourage him and

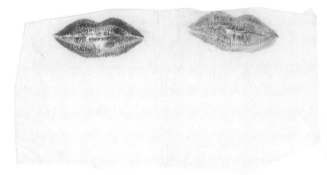

Opposite: Kevyn's first major cover, by Steven Meisel © 1984 *Rolling Stone* LLC. All rights reserved. Reprinted by permission.
Left: S.W.A.K.: Tina Turner's lip prints.

were kind of cool in the '80s, but she wanted red lipstick. Steven said, "If that's what she wants, let her have it. It's her signature. It makes her feel good,' " recalled Kevyn. "I started to understand that it wasn't about eyeliner and lipstick. It was about the way people feel."

He also realized that this glamorous new world wasn't the salvation he thought it would be. "When I put my head on the pillow that night, I still had the same childhood, the same emptiness that I'd felt

give him as much of the truth as I could."

Despite his personal struggles, Kevyn's career continued to take off. He was doing tons of editorial work, which traditionally pays very little, and subsidizing it with lucrative advertising assignments. (One day, for example, he'd make $70 working for Italian *Vogue,* and the next day he'd pull in $1,700 doing an ad for a company such as Geoffrey Beene, Barneys New York, or Capezio.) In 1985, he traveled outside the country for the first

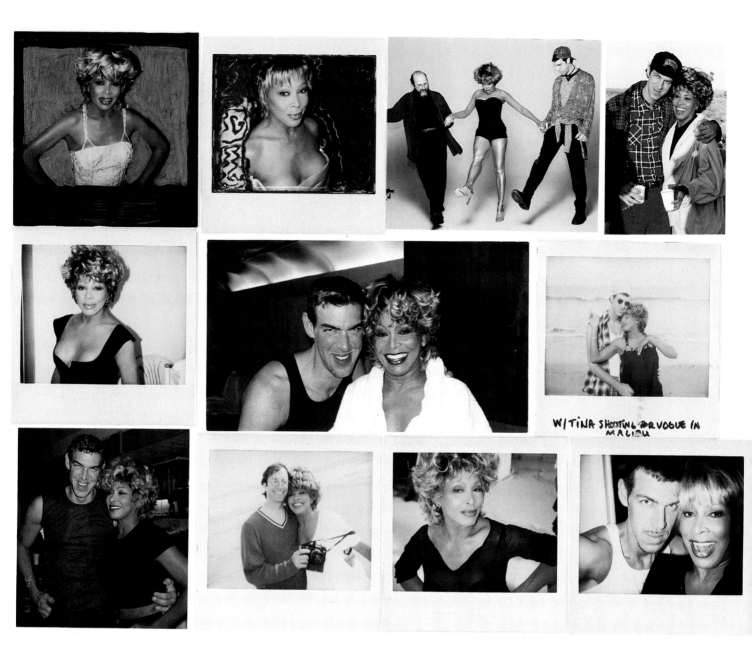

W/ TINA SHOOTING FOR VOGUE IN MALIBU

time for assignments in Barbados, Paris, and Monte Carlo. He was working with bigger celebrities and major photographers, from Jacqueline Bisset and Carly Simon to Bruce Weber, Arthur Elgort, Helmut Newton, and Annie Leibovitz. Kevyn was thrilled when Peter Lindbergh asked to photograph him for *L'Uomo Vogue,* the men's fashion magazine. Kevyn loved to pose for pictures and rarely left the set without a Polaroid of himself and the day's subject.

That summer, he marched in his very first Gay Pride Parade. "The people who outwardly admitted they were gay were few and far between back then," says Andrea Robinson. "But Kevyn was so up-front about being gay and having a boyfriend. It was a political statement without being a political statement." With the worst days of the AIDS epidemic and the accompanying rise in homophobia on the very near horizon, Kevyn's activism would take on a more serious tone.

In the years ahead, Kevyn would have a much larger audience for his message, which would evolve beyond tolerance to include issues of self-esteem and self-respect. No one knew it at the time, but the fashion industry was about to be

Vogue w/ Arthur Elgort
Beauty w/ Andrea Robinson
Hair: Christian

I ♥ NY NEW YORK
TRIP# 005421
07:55PM 07-09-85
MEDALLION# 6P22
DIST   1.80
FARE $ 2.80
FOR COMPLAINTS
869-4237

TIP 1⁰

CABfare
3.5⁰

MODELS: Christy
Claire Hoake
Bonnie Berman

s Armando

Mardi	Juillet
Dienstag	Juli
Martedi	Luglio · 190
Tuesday	July
Martes	Julio

9

Opposite: On assignment with Tina. First row, third picture: Michel Comte, Tina, and Kevyn. Bottom row, second picture: Herb Ritts and Tina.
Right: One of Kevyn's first assignments with Christy Turlington.

thrust onto a much bigger stage, and designers, models, editors, and makeup artists would become more recognizable than ever before.

The reason? Somebody had to satiate the public's desire for glamour, and many of Hollywood's hot new stars just weren't interested. "Things were different back then," says Julia Roberts. "Nobody even did my makeup the first time I went to the Oscars.

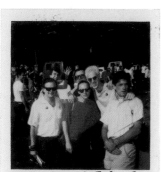

STEVEN, George, JED, ME + GAY PRIDE DAY 85' CLAUDE

If you had a seven o'clock premiere, you'd look at your watch at six-fifteen and say, 'Oh, God, I better go.' And you jumped in your car and went. There wasn't this hair, makeup, wardrobe thing that is commonplace now."

The media looked to the fashion world to fill the style void. Some of the faces that would help usher in this shift were just starting to appear in the magazines, such as a fifteen-year-old model from San Francisco named Christy Turlington and a certain fresh-faced teenager from Illinois with a very distinctive mole on her face.

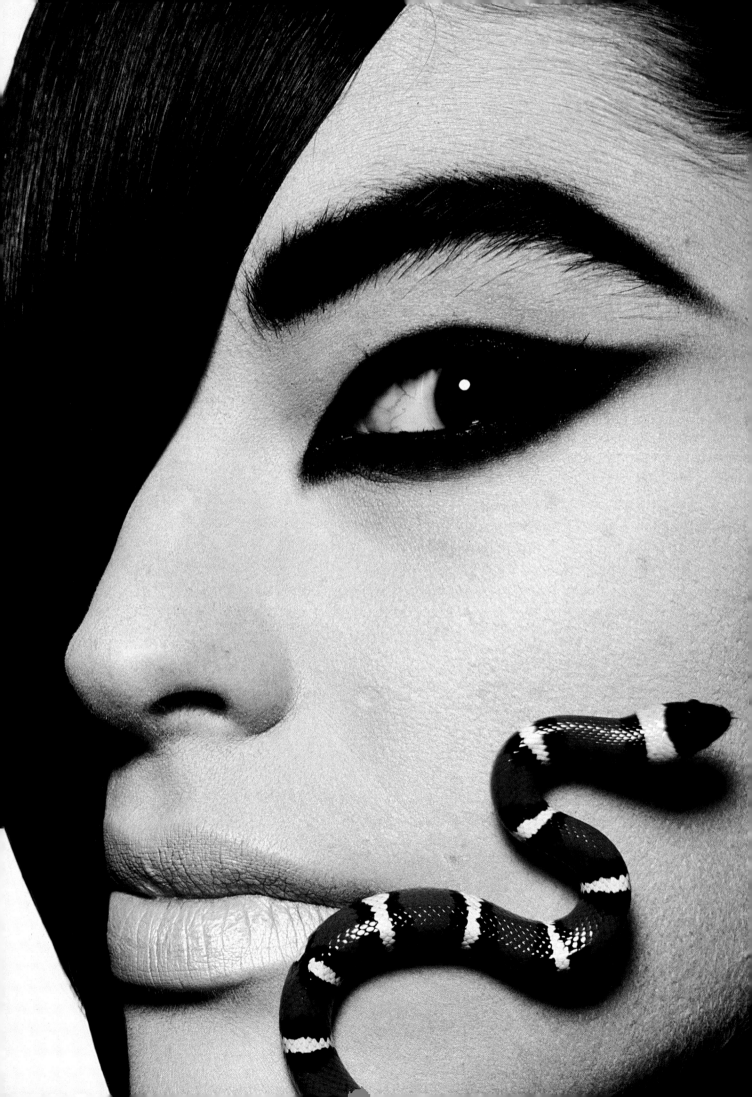

1986–1989

CHAPTER FOUR

THE COVER BOY YEARS

"I never went wrong by being myself."

There was no doubt that Kevyn had arrived. "He became the star of the moment really fast," says Andie MacDowell, the model-turned-actress whom Kevyn had befriended on a *New York Times* fashion shoot. Yet neither *Vogue* nor *Harper's Bazaar,* the two major American fashion magazines at the time, had bestowed its biggest honor on Kevyn: a cover.

Kevyn was desperate to work on one, but new talent rarely got a shot at something so prestigious. According to Polly Allen Mellen, then a fashion stylist at *Vogue,* the top photographers who worked on the covers tended to have a set team of stylists, hairdressers, and makeup artists they preferred. Breaking into those teams was difficult.

But not impossible. In late April, Kevyn's agent called to tell him that Richard Avedon had requested him for a *Vogue* cover shoot. At only twenty-four years old, Kevyn had come to the attention of the legendary fashion photographer.

For this shoot, the group included Polly, hairstylist Garren, and Estelle Lefebure, a curvy blond model from France. Garren says that Kevyn was awestruck when he walked into the studio. "He goes, 'I can't believe I'm here. I can't believe I'm

here.' I said, 'This is your moment, but just listen to what everyone says and follow along.'"

Things went well, because two weeks later Kevyn was booked for another Avedon session, this one with a young model named Cindy Crawford. The result was her very first *Vogue* cover. "It was such a big deal for both of us," says Crawford. "We worked together a lot after that. If I worked five days in a week, three or four of them were with Kevyn."

In 1986, Kevyn had four *Vogue* covers: July and October with Estelle, August with Cindy, and November with Paulina. Other work poured in as a result: Bill King and Bert Stern booked him to do *Mademoiselle* covers with such models as Monica Schnare, Alexa Singer, Michaela, and Jill Goodacre. There were German *Vogue* covers with Eric Boman, Italian *Vogue* covers with Hiro, and Versace ads with Avedon. In November, Kevyn finally got the chance to work with Francesco Scavullo, for a *Harper's Bazaar* shoot with model Pam Piper. "Kevyn was a perfectionist," says Scavullo. "I loved working with him because he knew what he was doing and he understood what I was doing."

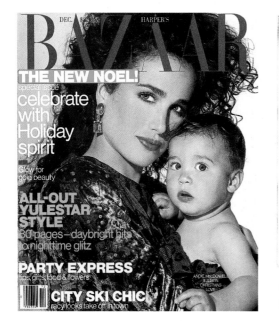

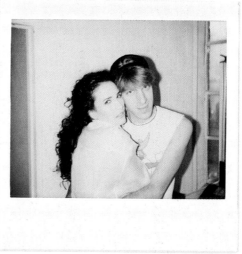

Left: Andie MacDowell and her son, Justin.
Right: Kevyn's early *Vogue* covers.

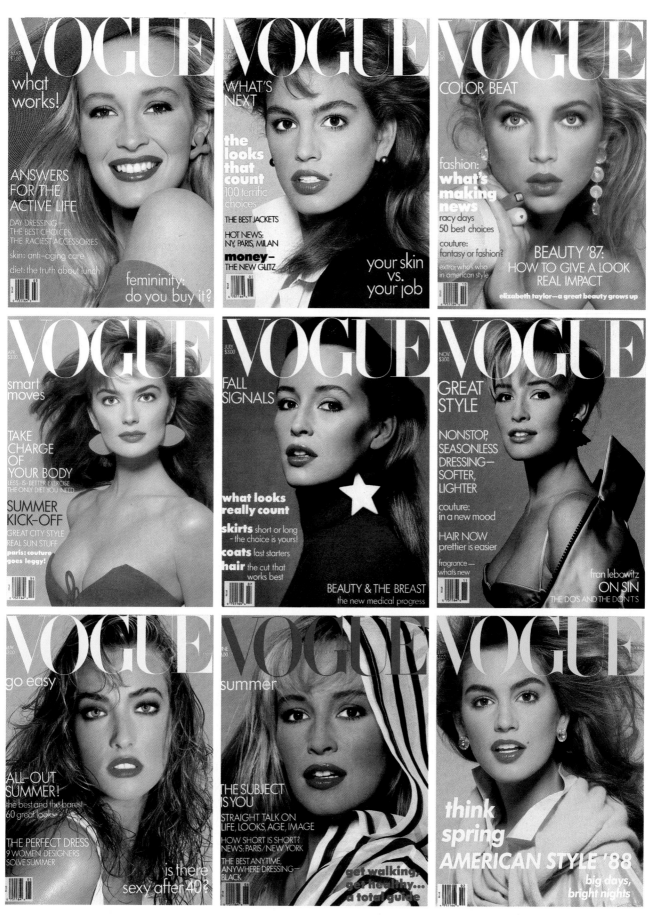

CATCHING UP WITH CINDY CRAWFORD

Kevyn and Cindy were two small-town kids who found fame and fortune in the big city. Their careers and reputations exploded around the same time as the supermodel phenomenon took off in the mid-'80s, making once nameless models and makeup artists recognizable personalities. They worked together on countless magazines shoots, covers, and advertising campaigns, helping cement Cindy's position as one of the most famous faces around. Kevyn admired not only her all-American good looks, but her tenacity and intelligence. "She's a real role model for models," wrote Kevyn. "She's as savvy as she is beautiful and was one of the first models to take charge of her career rather than leave it in the hands of someone else."

In turn, Cindy admired Kevyn for his individuality. "He never tried to be anyone other than who he was," she says. "He celebrated his differences. That's what was empowering about Kevyn. Not the makeup he put on your face, but how he lived his life and how true he was to himself." Here, Cindy reflects on Kevyn and their time together.

What was Kevyn's makeup like?

It was like a mask, but a beautiful mask. Kevyn totally erased your face and then he would start over. If anyone had come in the room after he had done foundation and nothing else, you literally couldn't see any features. You were a pair of nostrils. Then he would start building back. It was amazing. Kevyn almost painted the expression on your face. When makeup went toward a more natural look a few years later, I always felt that I didn't look like myself. I had gotten so accustomed to seeing Kevyn's makeup on my face.

Models are so used to putting makeup on and off and changing their look that I don't know if Kevyn's makeup was that emotional for us. But it was for some of the other women that he worked with. You could see just how much they relied on him for that "face." I think it gave them a certain kind of confidence.

Did Kevyn enjoy the ride?

One hundred percent. It was his whole life. He loved living in that fantasy world and working with women like Janet Jackson and Elizabeth Taylor and Liza Minnelli. That's why he was such a big star in his own right. He just lived it, breathed it. I love working with people like Kevyn who are so passionate. Even when they could do less of a job, they don't. It's like Herb Ritts. Herb chose to see the world at its most beautiful, and that's why everyone looked so great when Herb photographed them. That's how Kevyn was. He wanted everyone to be his vision of beauty.

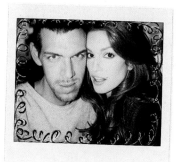 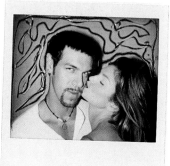 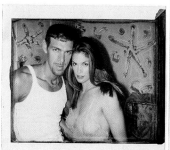 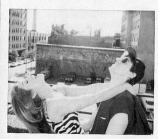

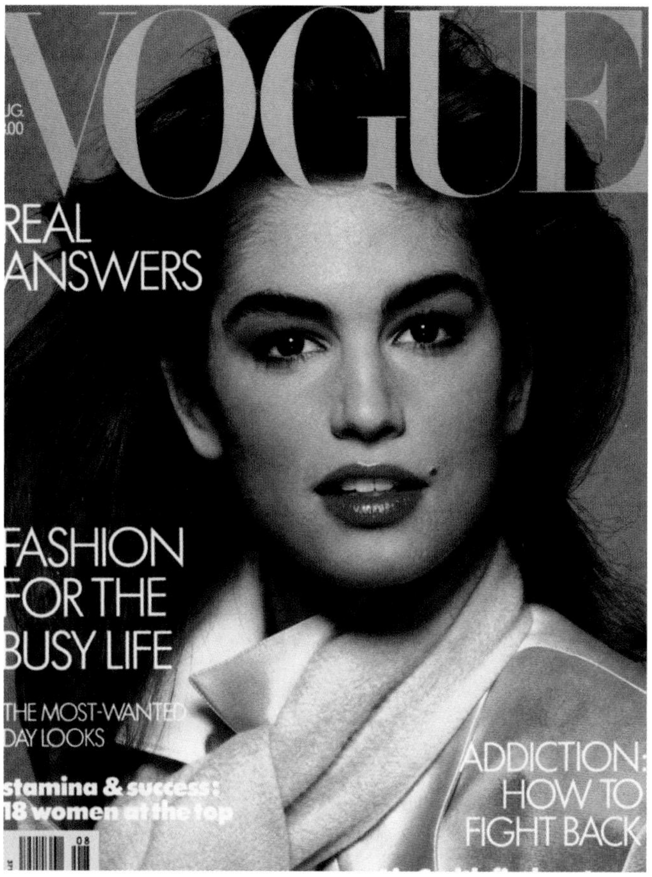

VOGUE

AUG.
$4.00

REAL
ANSWERS

FASHION
FOR THE
BUSY LIFE

THE MOST-WANTED
DAY LOOKS

stamina & success:
18 women at the top

ADDICTION:
HOW TO
FIGHT BACK

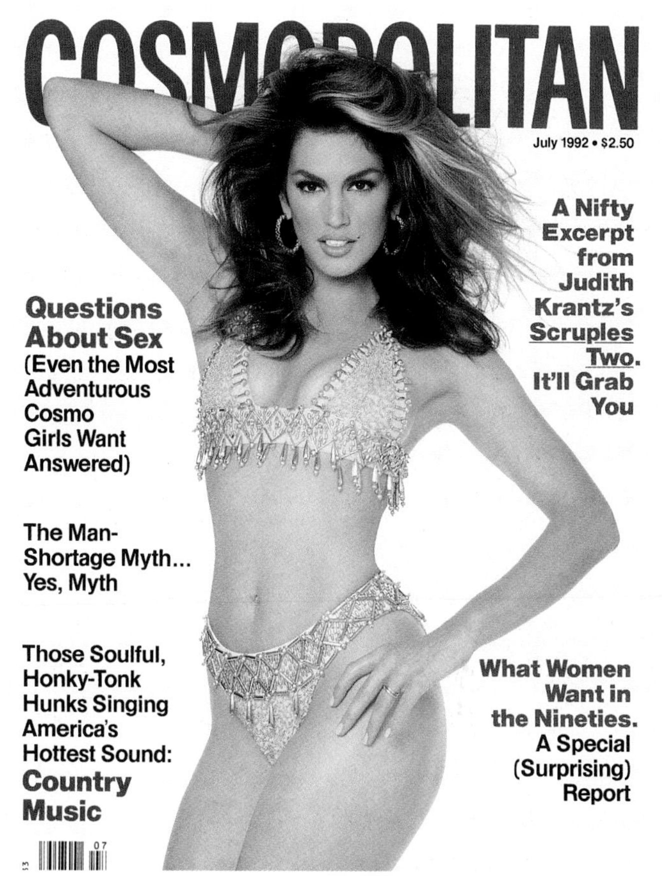

08

COSMOPOLITAN

July 1992 • $2.50

Questions About Sex (Even the Most Adventurous Cosmo Girls Want Answered)

The Man-Shortage Myth... Yes, Myth

Those Soulful, Honky-Tonk Hunks Singing America's Hottest Sound: **Country Music**

A Nifty Excerpt from Judith Krantz's <u>Scruples Two</u>. It'll Grab You

What Women Want in the Nineties. A Special (Surprising) Report

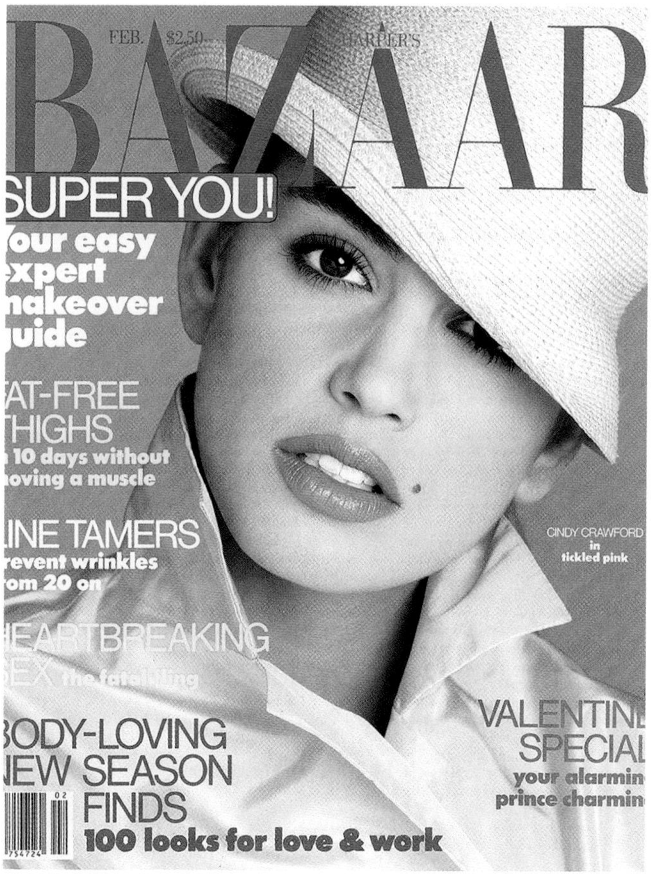

07

HARPER'S BAZAAR

FEB. $2.50

SUPER YOU!
Your easy expert makeover guide

FAT-FREE THIGHS
in 10 days without moving a muscle

LINE TAMERS
prevent wrinkles from 20 on

HEARTBREAKING
SEX the fatal thing

BODY-LOVING
NEW SEASON
FINDS
100 looks for love & work

CINDY CRAWFORD
in
tickled pink

VALENTINE
SPECIAL
your alarmin
prince charmin

02

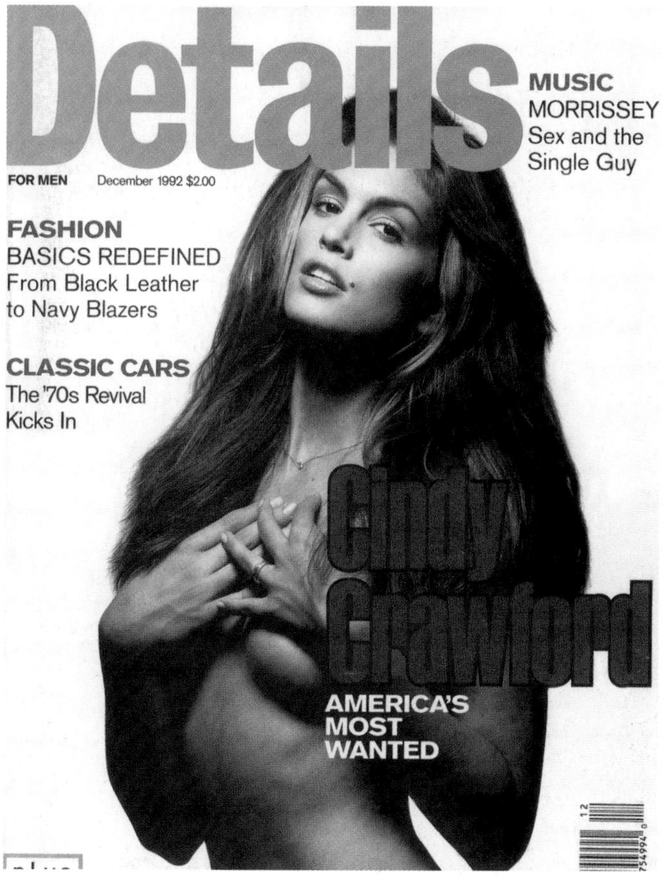

Details

FOR MEN   December 1992 $2.00

MUSIC
MORRISSEY
Sex and the
Single Guy

FASHION
BASICS REDEFINED
From Black Leather
to Navy Blazers

CLASSIC CARS
The '70s Revival
Kicks In

Cindy Crawford

AMERICA'S
MOST
WANTED

12

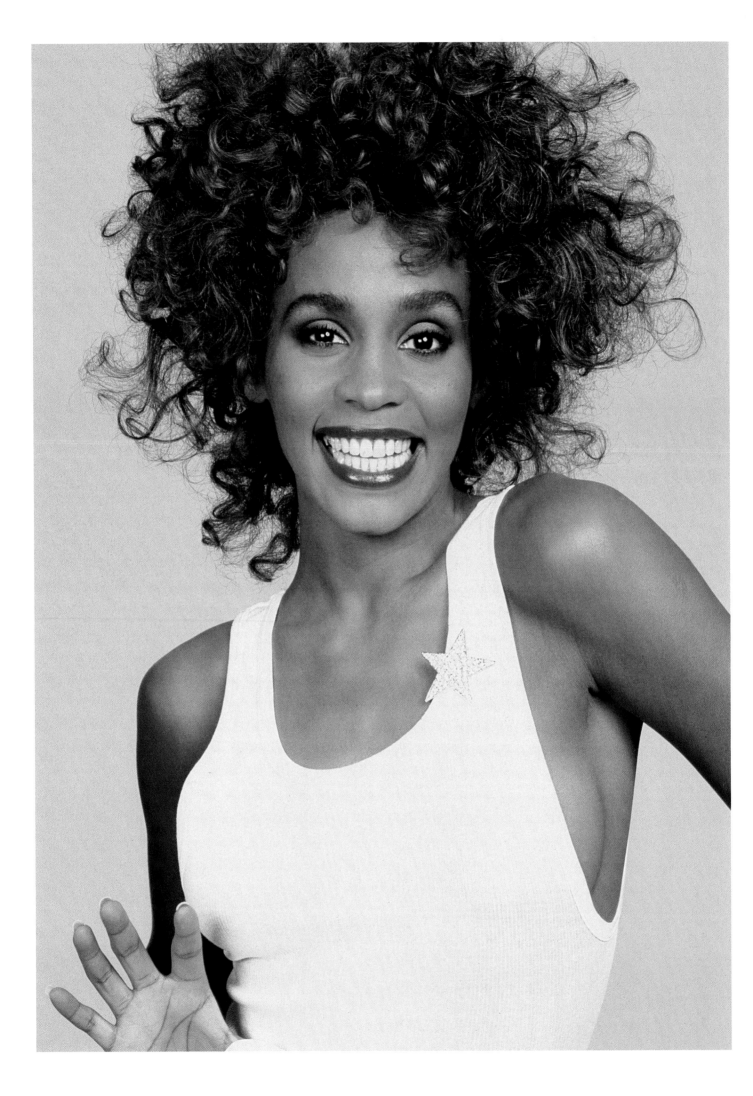

Kevyn especially hit it off with Irving Penn, the great photographer known for his masterful still-life pictures and intense portraits. Mr. Penn, as everyone called him, booked Kevyn time and time again for *Vogue* sittings and for prestigious advertising work with companies such as Chanel and L'Oréal. Kevyn later would say that he grew to love Penn like a grandfather.

To Andie MacDowell, the L'Oréal spokesmodel featured in those ads, it was obvious why the meticulous and professional Penn chose Kevyn. "Of course, Kevyn was a genius, but there's more to it than that," she says. "He knew how to handle himself. He knew that you show Mr. Penn respect. He

state of affairs is unfortunately not going to last forever. Doing a cover for *Glamour* is not going to hurt your career or 'image' one bit. Not doing it hurts you more in the long run. What I am trying to get across to you, in essence, is to please try to view your career beyond the September issue of *Vogue*."

Kevyn had a very distinct vision for his career, which included supermodels, celebrities, and haute couture. He hadn't spent all that time in Louisiana poring over fashion magazines and fantasizing about life in New York to work on straightforward jobs if he didn't have to.

His tactics paid off in 1987, his busiest year yet. He did seven consecutive *Vogue* covers,

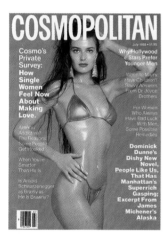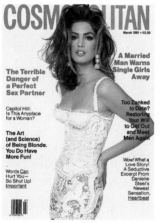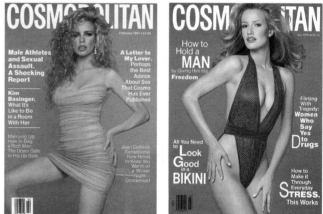

Left: Whitney Houston. Above: Some of Kevyn's *Cosmo* covers.

knew how to listen to the clients but at the same time be creative. A lot of people get freaked out by the pressure, but Kevyn never did. Or at least he never showed it."

Kevyn had switched agencies and was now represented by Helen Murray, who also handled hairdresser Maury Hopson and Kevyn's hero, Way Bandy. But Helen and Kevyn did not agree on the direction of Kevyn's career. "You are in the enviable position of having the privilege of picking your sittings," she wrote to him in a sharply worded letter. "This

from January through July, and Scavullo tapped him to do the iconic *Cosmopolitan* covers, famous for their cleavage, big hair, and bold makeup. Over the next few years, Kevyn transformed dozens of women, such as Kim Basinger and his friend Paulina Porizkova, into bombshell *Cosmo* Girls.

This was also the year in which Kevyn seriously "locked down," as Garren puts it, with some major celebrities. Each week he worked on another famous face for ads, magazines, awards shows, and more:

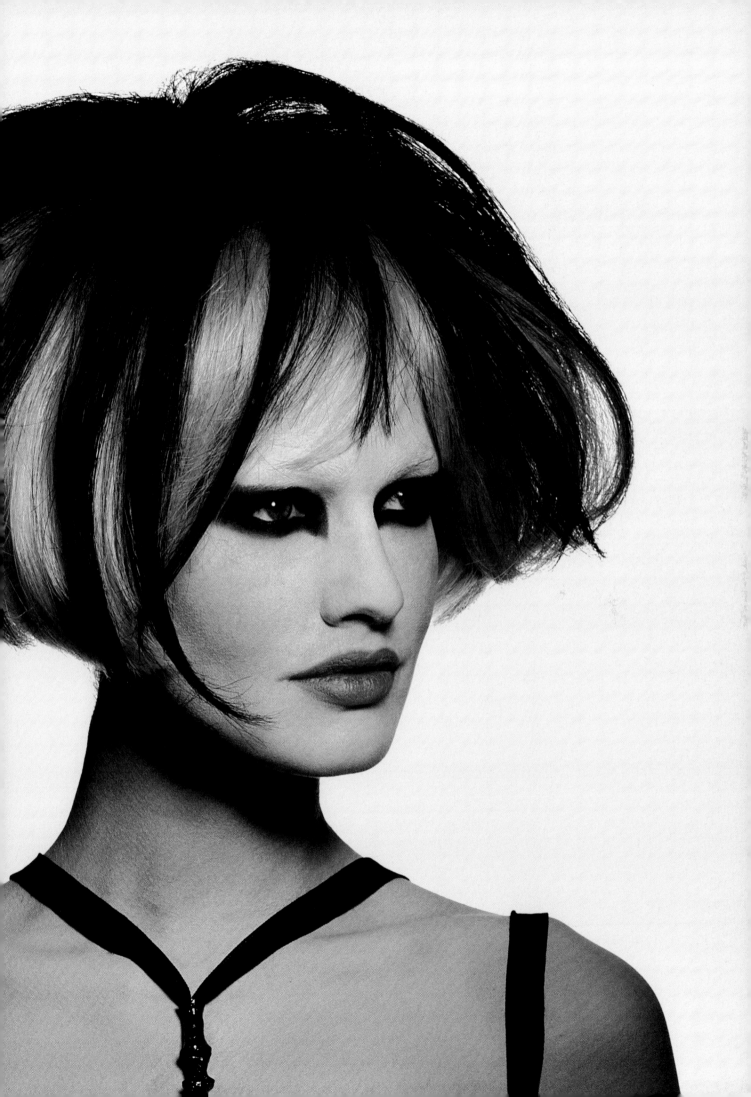

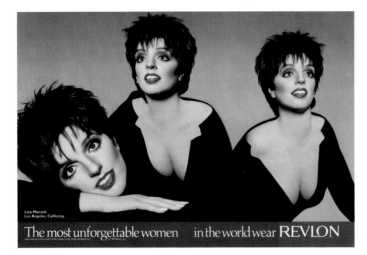

The most unforgettable women   in the world wear REVLON

Preceding spread: *Karen Mulder* by Irving Penn, New York
© 1992 Condé Nast Publications Inc.
Left: Liza Minnelli's Revlon ad by Avedon.
Opposite: Liza by Kevyn for "The Day After That," a single
she recorded to raise funds for the fight against AIDS.

Isabella Rossellini, Rosie Vela, Whitney Houston, and Debbie Harry were just a few. Even the icons started calling. Elizabeth Taylor, to his absolute delight, booked him three times in January alone. Mary Tyler Moore, whom Kevyn had grown up watching on TV, requested him for a public service announcement for what is now the Juvenile Diabetes Research Foundation. He did it for free and made a big impact on his idol. "I suspect that Kevyn helped every human being he came in contact with feel better about life and themselves," says Moore.

In February, Kevyn was introduced to a woman who would change his life: Liza Minnelli. Their first encounter was at a *Vanity Fair* shoot with Annie Leibovitz. In quick succession, he did her makeup for Carnegie Hall concert posters, a sitting with Victor Skrebneski, and her "The Most Unforgettable Women in the World Wear Revlon" campaign. Kevyn was drawn to survivors, so his connection with Minnelli was no surprise. Her reputation was that of a frail spirit, but she empowered Kevyn. She helped him understand the impact that his parents' drinking had on his life and brought him to his first ACOA (Adult Children of Alcoholics) meeting.

Kevyn described the two of them as best friends. "Makeup is such a personal thing that when you begin working regularly with someone who trusts you, you both open up and share your personal beliefs and philosophies," he later wrote. "That's the case with Liza and me. We're at the point where we finish each other's sentences and talk in Liza/Kevyn shorthand."

Although he was confronting some past pain, Kevyn remained very involved with his family. He was ecstatic over the arrival of the Aucoin clan's first grandchild, his niece and goddaughter Samantha Adkisson. Over the years, the two would become so close that Kevyn described her as his daughter. He also asked his parents to attend a convention for Parents, Families, and Friends of Lesbians and Gays (PFLAG) in Washington, D.C., with him. Isidore says it was the first time Kevyn really talked to him about being homosexual. "I had been in denial, I have to tell you," he says. "I never did question my love for Kevyn; it's just that I didn't want to believe he was gay."

When Isidore said he would go, Kevyn was shocked. Not only did Isidore and Thelma attend, but they were so inspired by the conference

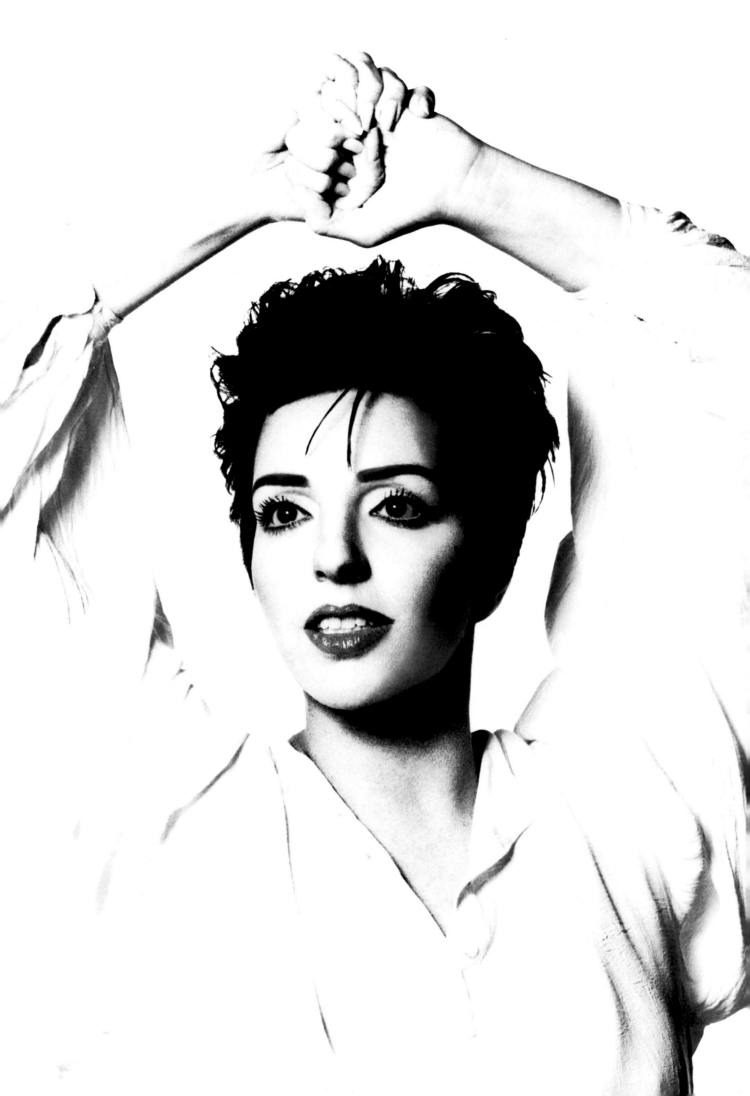

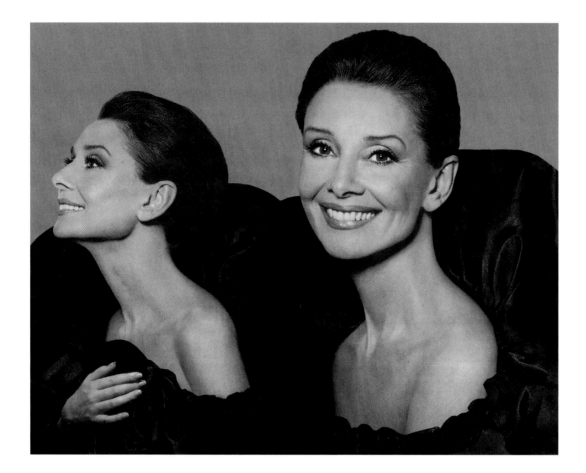

"I WAS SO NERVOUS THAT I HAD TO KEEP SAYING THE SERENITY PRAYER OVER AND OVER WHILE I WAS APPLYING AUDREY'S MAKEUP."

—KEVYN

Above: Audrey Hepburn's Revlon ad by Avedon.

that they formed a Lafayette chapter of the organization upon their return. They held meetings, published a newsletter, and even lobbied local politicians. Kevyn was amazed and touched by his parents' level of commitment, especially on the part of his father. "That he could come from the most racist, homophobic, misogynist background and still change makes me say to everyone out there, 'Don't underestimate your parents. Don't say they'll never understand,'" he said. "That's your arrogance."

By this time, Kevyn had become a true activist. He continued to march in New York's Gay Pride Parade every year, and he constantly spoke out about his homosexuality. Every time he was interviewed, which was happening with greater frequency, he mentioned his boyfriend Jed and the trouble faced by gay teens. Many in Kevyn's circle admired his stance. "He would take the subway to the studio wearing a long hot-pink coat!" says Sean Byrnes, the stylist on all the *Cosmo* covers. "I told him he was going to get killed, but he didn't care. He said, 'I'm gay, and I'm proud of it.' It was fantastic. What he did for gay rights and gay youth was extraordinary."

"I choose to live an open life, a life in which I can be proud of who I am, be happy about who I am, and let people know who I am," Kevyn told writer Katrinna Huggs for a story in his hometown newspaper. But things weren't that simple. By 1988, his career was everything he had hoped it would be, but his personal life wasn't. He barely had time for one. "He was bombarded with jobs," says Andie MacDowell. "It's irresistible when you have the opportunity to do such great work. You don't want to say no because you're afraid it's going to disappear, but he could have taken more time for himself."

Kevyn was too worried about his mother, who was recovering from a massive heart attack and triple-bypass surgery, to focus on himself. He worshipped his mother and was terrified that she might not make it. On top of this, his relationship with Jed was disintegrating. They broke up shortly after their six-year anniversary in February. Kevyn fell into such an emotional funk that he checked himself into the Suncoast Hospital in Largo, Florida. He later described it as a nervous breakdown and said the hospital stay was a way "to finally deal with all the things I had spent my life running from." He and Jed got back together later that year.

The day Kevyn returned from Florida, he was booked for another Revlon "Unforgettable Women" ad with Avedon, this time with one of his all-time favorite actresses, Audrey Hepburn. He had recuperated for two weeks before the shoot, but he still was rattled to meet the woman who was such a paragon of style and grace. "I was so nervous that I had to keep saying the serenity prayer over and over while I was applying Audrey's makeup," he wrote. "I really thought I was going to have go back to Suncoast."

Kevyn made an important connection that day with an up-and-coming designer named Isaac Mizrahi. "There was this immediate rapport and friendship between us," says Mizrahi, who had crafted a special black satin coat for Hepburn to wear in the ad. He remembers how awestruck they were dealing with Holly Golightly in the flesh. "Neither of us could believe it. We were, like, *'There she is in our midst.'* We were *dying.*"

Around this time, Kevyn got a call from Andrea Robinson, the *Vogue* editor who gave him his start. She was now president of Ultima II and wanted to develop a cosmetics line based on natural colors. Since Kevyn's favorite palette for the face included beiges, sandy pinks, taupes, choco-

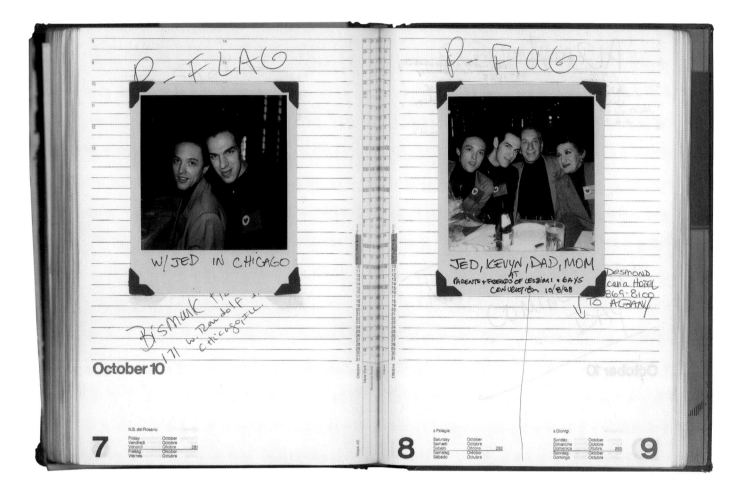

P-FLAG

P-FIAG

W/ JED IN CHICAGO

BISMARK #12
W. Randolf
CHICAGOPILL
10/71

JED, KEVYN, DAD, MOM
AT
PARENTS + FRIENDS OF LESBIANS + GAYS
CONVENTION 10/8/88

DESMOND
cana HOTEL
869-8100
TO ALBANY

October 10

7 | N.S. del Rosario
Friday
Vendredi
Venerdì
Freitag
Viernes | October
Octobre
Ottobre
Oktober
Octubre | 281

8 | s Pelagia
Saturday
Samedi
Sabato
Samstag
Sábado | October
Octobre
Ottobre
Oktober
Octubre | 282

9 | s Dionigi
Sunday
Dimanche
Domenica
Sonntag
Domingo | October
Octobre
Ottobre
Oktober
Octubre | 283

lates, and other flattering, feminine neutrals, he jumped when Robinson asked him to help perfect the shades for the collection.

The result was called The Nakeds. It was all about no-makeup makeup, and the tagline was "Look Like Yourself, Only Better." Women had never seen colors like this compiled in a single collection. "At a time when makeup was still stuck in the disco, Kevyn brought it into broad daylight," wrote Linda Wells, the editor in chief of *Allure,* years later.

The Nakeds was one of the biggest successes the industry had ever experienced. "We couldn't even fill the orders we had," recalls Robinson. "It was just this massive explosion we never expected. We had every person in Hollywood calling for product."

Buoyed by the experience, Robinson and Kevyn considered doing a Kevyn Aucoin makeup collec-

tion. "We talked about it before any of those makeup artist lines came out," says Robinson. "We got to the point where we discussed it with a lawyer, but we never moved forward." It would be more than a decade before Kevyn launched products under his own name.

At the end of 1988, Kevyn went home to spend the holidays with his family and to see Samantha, who was now an adorable toddler with blond hair, big gray-blue eyes, and mile-long lashes. In the back of his datebook, he scribbled a list of celebrities he hoped to work with in the year ahead. Kevyn loved people who could make him laugh, and the names reflected that: Carol Burnett, Bette Midler, Tracey Ullman, Catherine O'Hara, and Andrea Martin. Topping the list, of course, was his beloved Barbra Streisand.

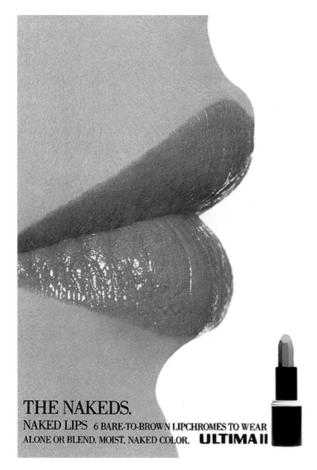

THE NAKEDS.
NAKED LIPS 6 BARE-TO-BROWN LIPCHROMES TO WEAR
ALONE OR BLEND. MOIST, NAKED COLOR. **ULTIMA II**

In 1989, Kevyn moved to Jed's new agency, Root-McKenna, and continued to get a dizzying number of assignments. Christy Brinkley, Diana Ross, teen pop sensation Debbie Gibson, Barbara Walters, and Shirley MacLaine ("She liked Kevyn's makeup so much she actually slept in it," says Scavullo) were a few of the stars he met that year. He worked for British *Vogue* for the first time, with Steven Klein, and he partnered quite a bit with Matthew Rolston, the photographer who is now a successful music video director. "Kevyn had such a gift," says Rolston. "It wasn't just about the makeup. It was about love and affection. He had a true interest in the people he worked with and about what would work for them."

This kindness even extended to the assistants, both his and the photographers'. "Kevyn would always hang out with us during lunch and tell jokes, give massages, and crack our backs," says Billy Jim, a photographer who used to assist Irving Penn.

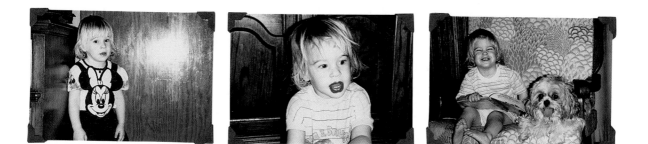

"I remember Mr. Penn shaking his head at us one time when we ordered pizza and McDonald's french fries in Paris. Kevyn was like a big brother to me."

He even helped Michael Thompson get his start. Thompson, who also was assisting Penn when he and Kevyn met, was eager to start his own photography career. Kevyn helped by recommending him for jobs at major magazines. "When Kevyn believed in someone, he fought for them," says Thompson, who today shoots the covers for *W* and *Allure.* "He was very generous that way."

"When Kevyn was doing the fashion shows, there would always be a Kiehl's goodie bag for each of the assistants," says makeup artist Charlie Green, who worked backstage with Kevyn on everything from Ralph Lauren presentations to a Vivienne Westwood show at the Lido in Paris. "It was a little gesture, but he always made sure there was something for everyone."

Kevyn continued to spend a lot of time with Liza Minnelli. His datebook was filled with entries like "dinner with Liza," "movies with Liza," and "shopping with Liza." He worked on her *Results* album cover with David LaChapelle and did her makeup for the Grammys, Arsenio Hall's talk show, and her video "Don't Drop Bombs." She took him to dinner at Frank Sinatra's house in Los Angeles and to Hal-

ston's apartment in Manhattan. The famed fashion designer, who was dying of AIDS at the time, took Kevyn aside and whispered, "Take care of my Liza." Halston passed away a few months later.

With Minnelli's support, Kevyn talked to his parents about their drinking. He convinced Thelma to start attending Al-Anon meetings, but Isidore said he would quit on his own, which he did. During difficult times, Kevyn often turned to a book called *One Day at a Time in Al-Anon,* a tiny volume meant to help the reader "find in each day a measure of comfort, serenity and a sense of achievement," according to an introductory passage. "It discourages dwelling on past errors and disappointments; visualizes the future only as a series of new days, each a fresh opportunity for self-realization and growth."

On August 7, 1989, Kevyn took an extra copy and inscribed it to his father. He wrote, "Dear Daddy, This little book has helped me tremendously to cope with my problems—to see the positive—and to reexamine myself. I hope you will find it as helpful as I have! I love you, Kevyn."

For whatever reason, Kevyn never gave Isidore the book. Instead, Isidore found it on a bookshelf in Kevyn's apartment after his death. He brought it home to Lafayette and still reads a passage from it every day.

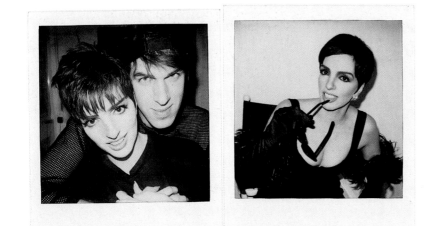

Left: Kevyn and Liza.
Opposite: Christy, Liza, Kevyn, and Steven Meisel at a party in Kevyn's honor at the Roxy. Photo by Roxanne Lowit.

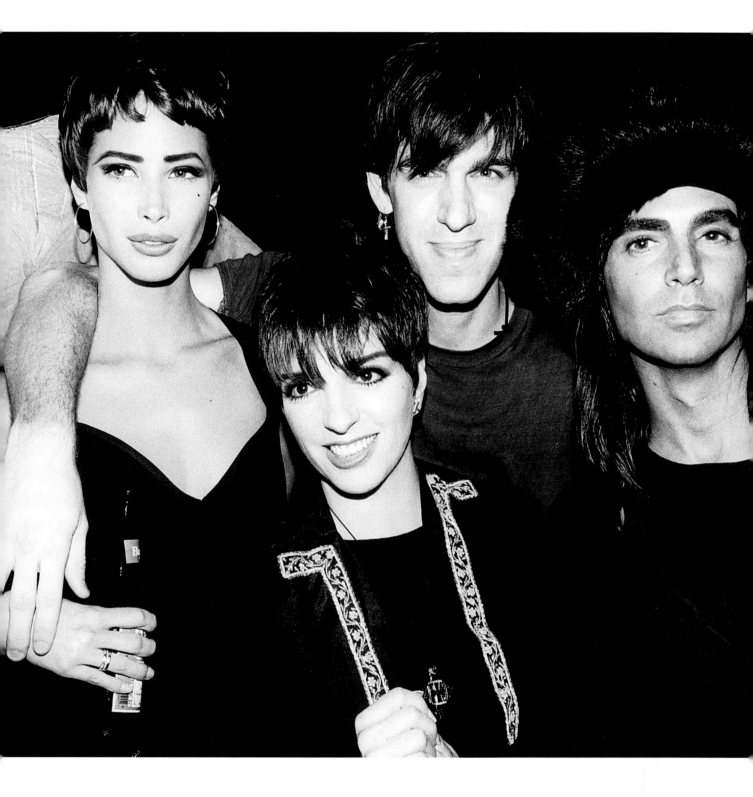

"If you wait your whole life for somebody else to tell you it's okay

1990–1994

CHAPTER FIVE

THE SUPER YEARS

allure

PERFECT MAKEUP
(No Kidding)

GLITTERING FASHION

Best Bodies In America

THE KING OF HAIR COLOR TELLS ALL

The Search for Smoother Skin

REDHEAD ALERT!

Inside Fragrance
Plus Who Wears What and Why

BEAUTY GUIDE
Hot Haircutters
Tipping Tip Sheet

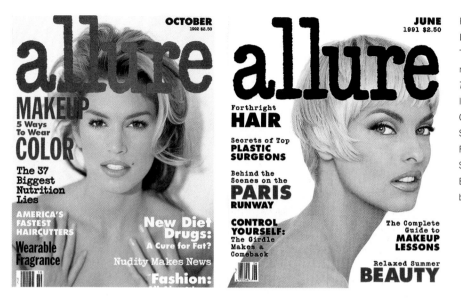

Preceding spread: Kevyn and Linda Evangelista mobbed at a Todd Oldham show; Bill Cunningham, legendary lensman for *The New York Times*, smiles at left. Photo by Eric Sakas. Opposite and left: Linda by Steven Meisel. Far left: Cindy Crawford by Sante D'Orazio. Below: Kevyn and his new boyfriend, Donald Reuter.

Kevyn and his boyfriend Jed broke up for good in 1990. Together they had built lives and careers they never imagined, yet they had grown apart. The two remained friends, and Jed continued to represent Kevyn as his agent. This was a pattern Kevyn would repeat in the years ahead: While most lovers move on when they part ways, Kevyn's serious boyfriends remained part of his inner circle.

Careerwise, Kevyn was as hot as ever, and his rates were among the highest in the industry. "I'd look better if Kevyn Aucoin weren't so damned expensive," quipped Joan Rivers.

That summer, Kevyn got a call from his friend Linda Wells, whom he had met when she was an assistant in *Vogue*'s beauty department. Wells had been named editor of a new Condé Nast magazine and wanted to take Kevyn to lunch at Le Cirque to discuss the venture. "Jackie O sat at a table near the door, eating asparagus with her fingers," Wells later wrote. "Ivana Trump and a pack of blondes carried on at a table next to Robin Leach. Kevyn studied the menu and made a face. Then he asked the waiter for spaghetti with butter, ketchup on the side, and a glass of Coca-Cola. Kevyn had few pretensions."

The new magazine was called *Allure.* Set to launch in spring 1991, it would have all the style and sophistication of *Vogue,* but its raison d'être was beauty, not fashion. To Kevyn, it sounded like a dream come true. In October, he was named contributing editor, a move that would position him as more than just a behind-the-scenes player.

That fall, Kevyn *finally* met Barbra Streisand. Scavullo had been hired to photograph her and Nick Nolte for the poster of their upcoming movie, *The Prince of Tides,* and Kevyn was booked to be on the set—but only for touchups. "In all the years of making movies and everything, I've always done my own makeup," explains Streisand. "When I was eighteen, a friend of mine who was an actual artist taught me how to do my face in terms of light and shadow, so I've been doing it ever since."

Kevyn, who never got tongue-tied around anyone, was so flustered that day he could barely speak. He returned home to Donald Reuter, his boyfriend at the time, disappointed by his lim-

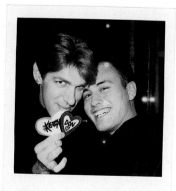

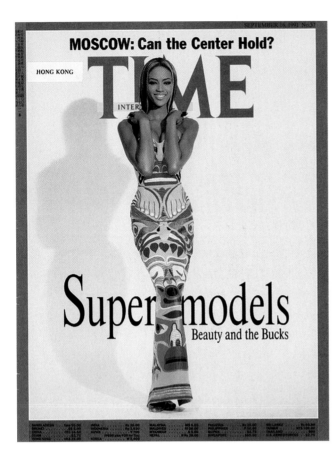

Left: Naomi Campbell by Brigitte Lacombe for *Time* magazine.
Opposite: Audrey Hepburn by Steven Meisel for *Vanity Fair*
© Condé Nast Publications Inc.

ited role at the shoot and mad at himself for not telling Streisand what she had meant to him.

The next year, 1991, Kevyn teamed up again with Steven Meisel, the photographer who had helped establish his career in the early '80s. They worked on dozens of assignments, including a radiant *Vanity Fair* cover of Audrey Hepburn. Hepburn liked Kevyn so much that she started booking him for personal appearances. Jed remembers getting the phone calls from Switzerland, where Hepburn lived, and hearing that distinctive voice on the other end. "That's a true star," says Jed. "Somebody who doesn't have the assistant of an assistant of an assistant make the call."

If Hepburn represented old-guard glamour, then Linda, Christy, Naomi, and company represented the new. *Time* magazine took notice of the phenomenon with a cover story titled "Supermodels," featuring Naomi Campbell in a Todd Oldham totem-pole dress and, of course, Kevyn Aucoin makeup.

"They're everywhere," reported *Time.* "Super-models are always perfectly coiffed and coutured, manicured and made up," in comparison to "movie stars who dress down in blue jeans and prefer environmental preservation to nightclubbing."

If anything captured the essence of that era, it was the Meisel pictures of Linda Evangelista with makeup by Kevyn and hair by Garren. The quartet was fashion's dream team. Editors and advertisers knew they had a hit on their hands when those four got together. "There were so many memorable sittings we did with Linda," says Garren, who famously took the model blond, red, and back to brunet. "The *Allure* covers, Italian *Vogue.* Kevyn made her look so amazing in all those photographs."

Kevyn started out 1992 with a block of Scavullo bookings, including one assignment he normally might have turned down: a *Ladies Home Journal* cover. But he accepted because the subject was the wise-cracking, irreverent comedian Roseanne.

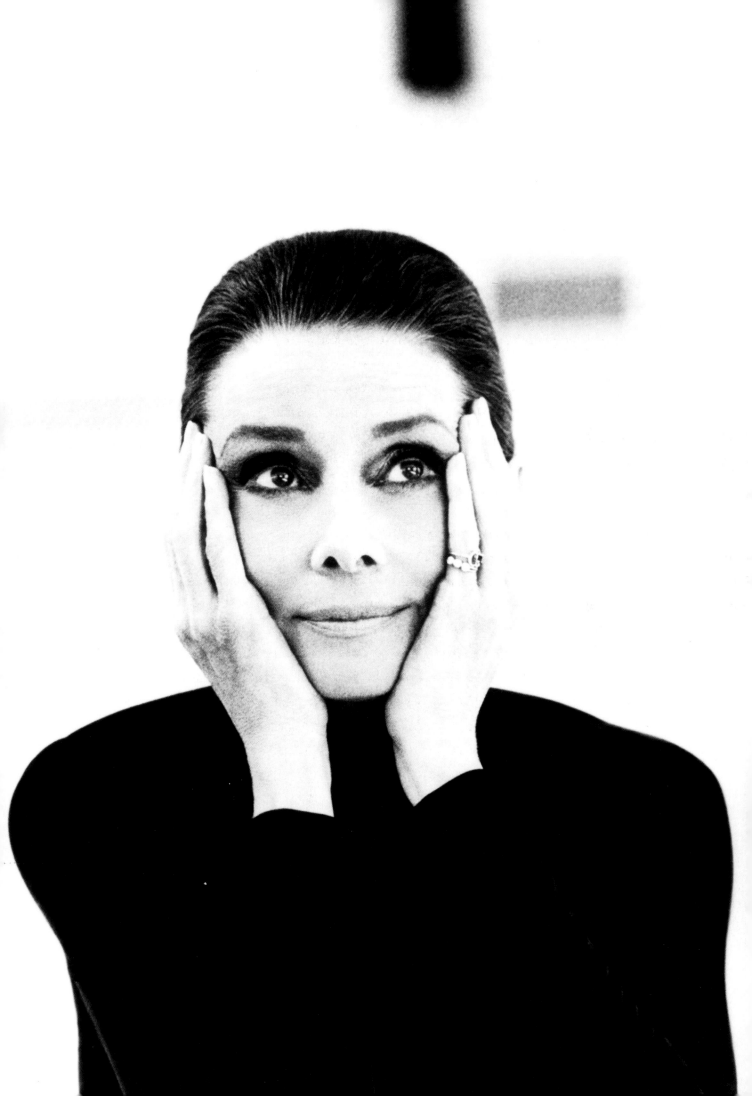

Below: Kevyn and Linda. Bottom: Kevyn and Roseanne. Opposite: Linda by Steven Meisel © 1991 Italian *Vogue*. Courtesy of Condé Nast Publications Inc.

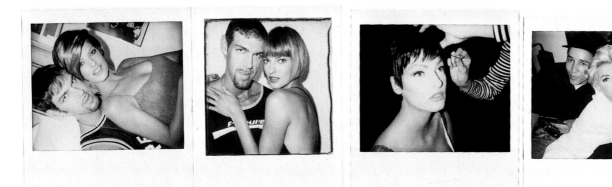

Kevyn and Scavullo went for full-throttle glamour, and Kevyn completely resculpted Roseanne's face with makeup. The result was a total departure both for the magazine and for Roseanne, who was mad for her new look and Kevyn. "I knew I had met my best friend in all the world—another small-town guy who hated artifice, even though he lived it, like me," says Roseanne. "He made me gorgeous for Scavullo, and we ate about two hundred cookies while doing that one."

In February, Kevyn got some devastating news. Jay Theall, his cousin and earliest confidant, had died of AIDS. Jay's partner, Robert, had succumbed to the disease only the month before. As teenagers, Kevyn and Jay had dreamed of running away to New York, where they would be rich and famous and party with the jet set. Instead, Jay stayed behind and worked as a hairdresser in Lake Charles, Louisiana. "I always figured things might have been a little different for Jay if he had followed Kevyn," says Jay's mother, Laura Bourgeois.

As Jay was dying, Kevyn had tried to keep his spirits up with cards, phone calls, and presents. "You were the first person I told I was gay," wrote Kevyn in one of his notes. "You were the first person to accept me as I am. You are in my heart forever." Jay especially loved the Chinese pajamas that Kevyn sent while he was in the hospital. "The nurses and I put them on Jay and walked him around the hall so he could show them off to everyone," recalls Laura.

Kevyn couldn't get back to Louisiana in time for the funeral, but he did manage to pay his last respects. "I went to Jay's grave one day, and there were three American Beauty roses, real ones, stuck in the ground," says Laura. "I always suspected it was Kevyn who put them there. There was no one else who would have done that."

That summer, two important names appeared in Kevyn's datebook for the first time: Gilles Bensimon, the head photographer and publication director of *Elle* magazine, and photographer Patrick Demarchelier. Kevyn paired with Bensimon on

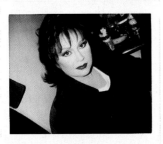
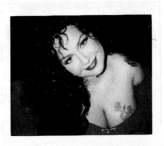
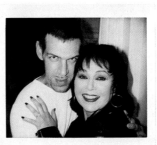
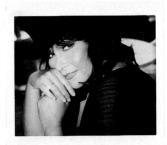

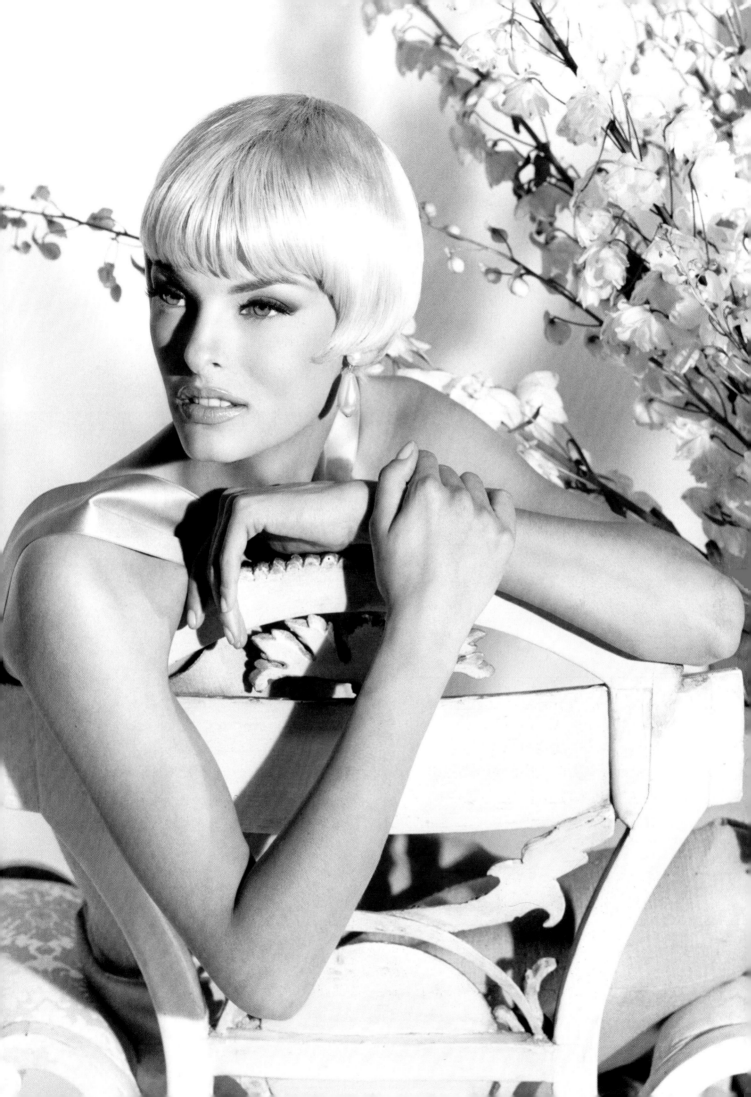

shoots featuring Whitney Houston, Naomi Campbell, and the new model on the block, Beverly Peele.

At the same time, Kevyn and Demarchelier were busy with the relaunch of *Harper's Bazaar.* Liz Tilberis, the former British *Vogue* editor, had been brought to New York to give the publication an injection of elegance and excitement. Her hop across the pond was the biggest thing to happen to fashion magazines since Anna Wintour shook up *Vogue* four years earlier, so the industry was abuzz with anticipation. Kevyn would play a big role in the Tilberis era of *Bazaar,* doing dozens of shoots and covers with fashion directors Paul Cavaco and Tonne Goodman before Tilberis tragically succumbed to ovarian cancer.

Kevyn, meanwhile, was dealing with a personal issue that had obsessed him for years: he wanted to find his birth mother. Thelma and Isidore Aucoin always were upfront with their four children about their adoptions, but the identities of their birth parents were a mystery. All the children's records had been sealed, since adoption was such a secretive process in the 1960s. "Kevyn thought about it every day," says Donald Reuter. "He had tried so many avenues to locate his birth mother, but they were all dead ends."

Then, one day, a friend put him in touch with a woman who promised to find his mother for a substantial fee. Less than two weeks later, Kevyn had his birth mother's name and phone number. On October 5, 1992, he nervously placed the call and spoke to Nelda Mae Sweat for the very first time.

"I said, 'Oh, my God, is it really you?' " recalls Nelda. "He said, 'It's really me,' and I cried and cried and cried." Nelda was married and living in Louisiana with her husband, John T. Williams, and her two sons, Kevin and Keith, who, in a freakish coincidence, happened to have the same exact names Thelma Aucoin gave her two sons. Nelda's family knew about the child from her past, so they weren't stunned when Kevyn made contact.

Below: Beverly Peele and Naomi by Gilles Bensimon for *Elle*. Opposite: Some of Kevyn's *Bazaar* covers.

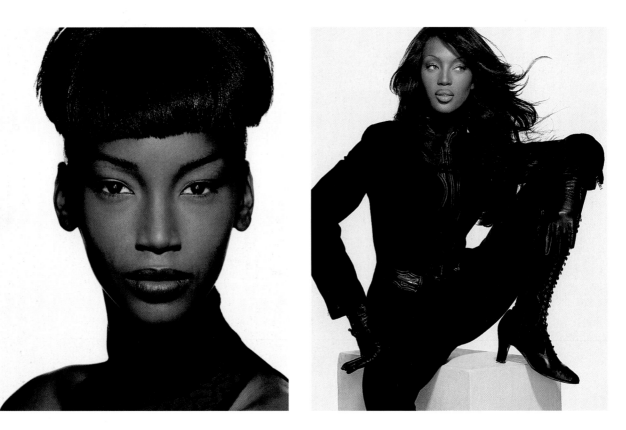

Harper's BAZAAR

MARCH $ 3.00

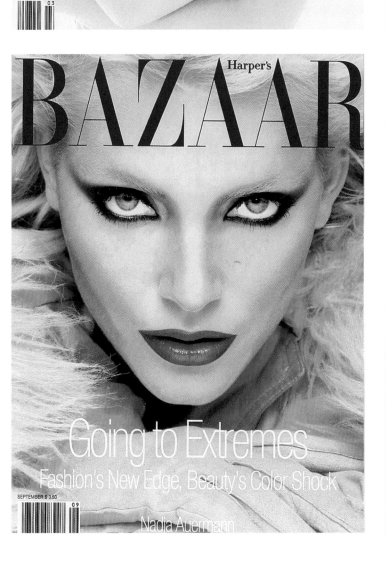

Next: It's Short & Sexy, Sensuous Knits, Wild Colors, Dreamy Dresses. Hard or Soft Fitness
Meryl Streep: Margaritas, Movies, and Her Life
Avedon's One Man Show: The Bazaar Years

03

Harper's BAZAAR

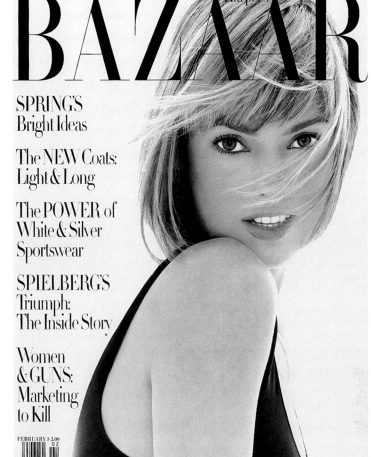

SPRING'S Bright Ideas

The NEW Coats: Light & Long

The POWER of White & Silver Sportswear

SPIELBERG'S Triumph: The Inside Story

Women & GUNS: Marketing to Kill

FEBRUARY $ 3.00

02

BAZAAR Harper's

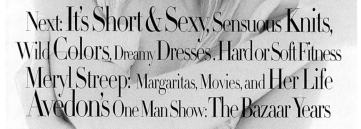

Going to Extremes
Fashion's New Edge, Beauty's Color Shock

SEPTEMBER $ 3.50

09

Nadja Auermann

BAZAAR Harper's

Winter Dressing Paris Couture Redford Coppola

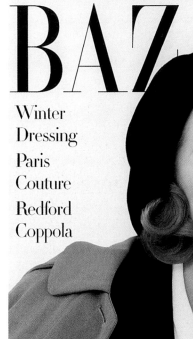

OCTOBER $ 3.00

10

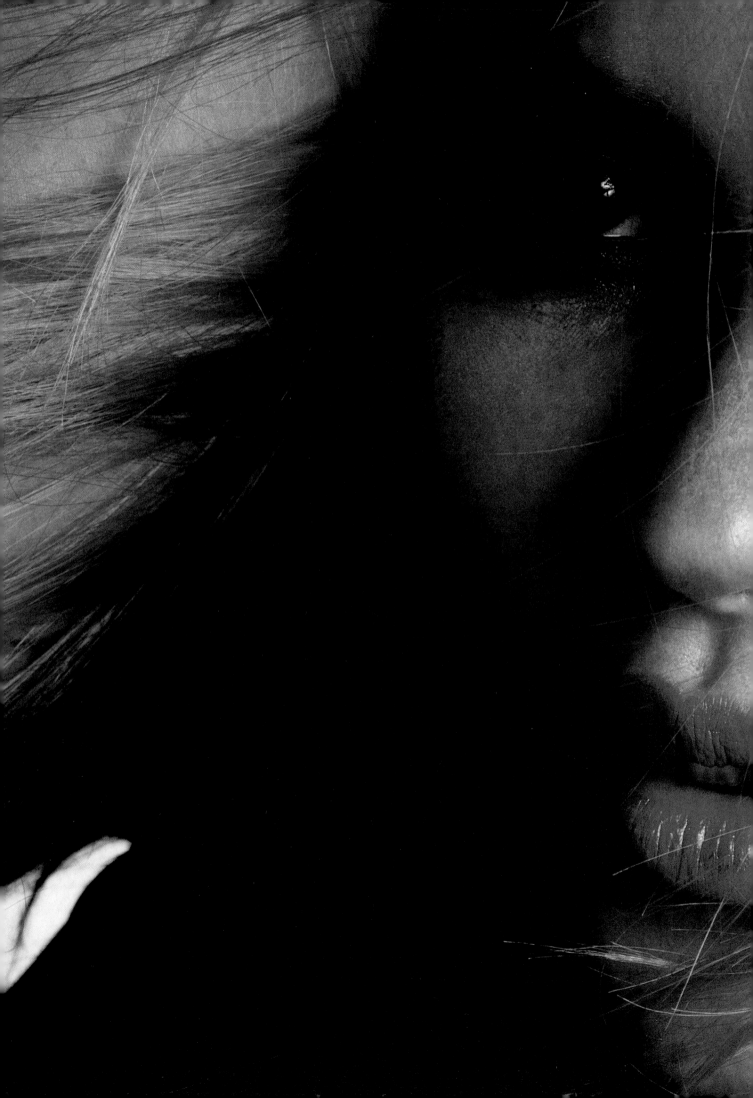

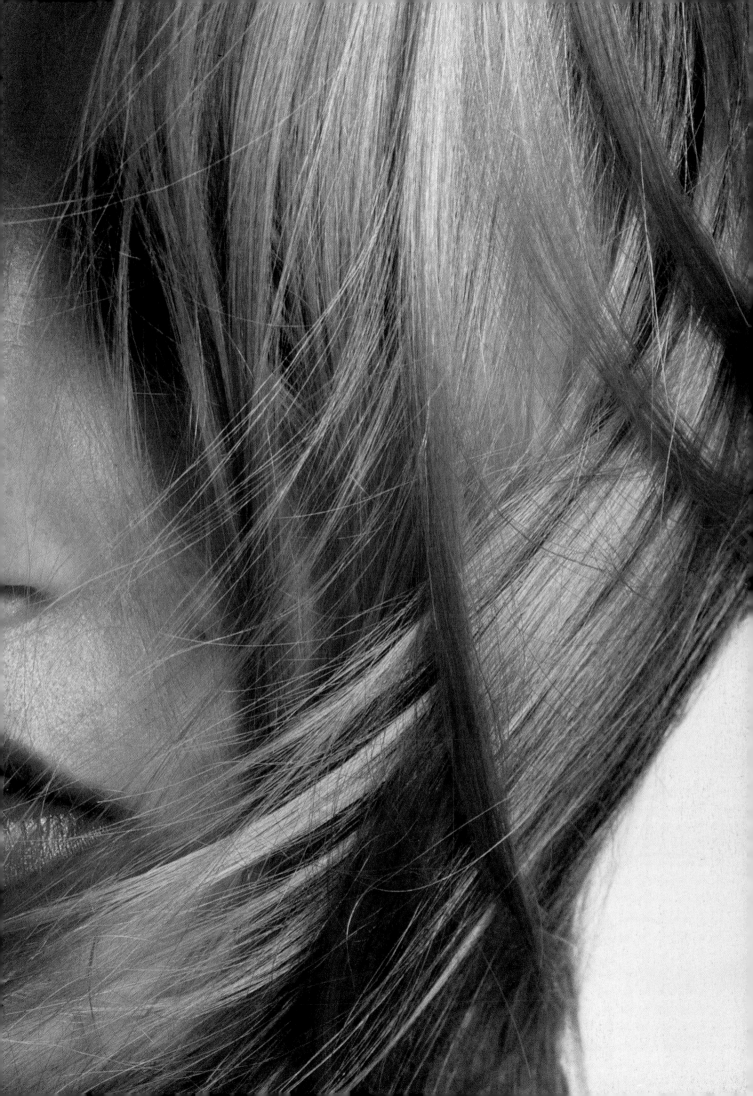

Nelda told Kevyn that his father was Jerry Burch, a refinery worker living in Baton Rouge with his wife and two daughters. Kevyn found his phone number and called him directly. "Kevyn was real nervous, asking me all sorts of questions, so I finally said, 'Who are you, and why are you wanting to know all this?'" recalls Jerry. "That's when Kevyn said, 'I think you're my dad.' I was shocked." Jerry says that Nelda had told him the baby was his, but he didn't believe her. As a result, he and Kevyn agreed that a paternity test should be performed. (It later showed that Kevyn was indeed his son.)

Nelda and Kevyn decided they would meet at Thanksgiving, when Kevyn was home for the holidays. She quickly sent him a letter to say everything she hadn't said over the phone. "Please forgive me for thirty lost years," she wrote. "We will never be able to make it up, but there is love here."

Kevyn shared his big news with all his friends. He read Nelda's letter to Brana Wolf, a well-known fashion stylist, while on break during an assignment in L.A. "We went up to the roof of the Four Seasons Hotel, and he told me the whole family history," says Wolf. "He was so excited." Donna Karan says that Kevyn felt "complete" because of his discovery. "He was so ecstatic that chills went up your spine," says the designer. "It's not that he didn't love his family. He adored them, but he needed to resolve where he came from."

When he finally met Nelda, it was an emotional, tear-filled reunion. Nelda went through her family tree, and Kevyn told her stories about his upbringing. They laughed over their mutual fondness for rabbits. At Christmas, Kevyn met Jerry and his fam-

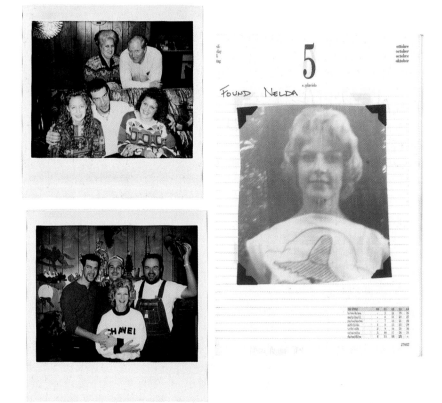

Preceding spread: Kate Moss by Nick Knight © British *Vogue* / Condé Nast Publications Ltd. Above left: Kevyn with his birth parents and siblings. Above right: Kevyn's datebook from the day he found his birth mother.

ily. "Kevyn's life was a total flip side of mine, but we got along really well," says Jerry. "He was full of life, always wanting to learn, and he loved people. We had that in common."

But there was one part of his life they couldn't accept. Both Nelda and Jerry were opposed to homosexuality. Today his birth parents say they loved Kevyn despite his sexual orientation. "I'm not saying that I don't love Kevyn for who he is," says Nelda, "because I do." As for Jerry, "my religious and personal feelings on the subject had nothing to do with our relationship. He was my child," he says, his voice breaking. "You love them for who they are."

In the midst of this was New York Fashion Week. Oscar de la Renta and Geoffrey Beene had been booking Kevyn for their shows for years, and this season, Todd Oldham, Ralph Lauren, Katherine Dionos, Isaac Mizrahi, and Perry Ellis followed suit. The designers were becoming stars themselves, and with those famous supermodels parading down their catwalks, who better to have backstage than beauty's biggest name?

Since there were more than a dozen models in each show, Kevyn would bring several assistants to get the job done. "But all the girls wanted Kevyn," remembers Oldham. "Cindy, Naomi, Christy, and Kate would be lined up behind him, waiting. He would manage to do sixteen, seventeen, eighteen girls himself. Not just one time but every single show." The supermodel backup meant that shows started late. "It was kind of a nightmare, but you needed someone with his authority," says Mizrahi. "If Kevyn did your makeup, you felt made up. You

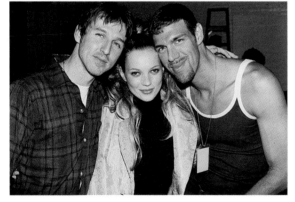

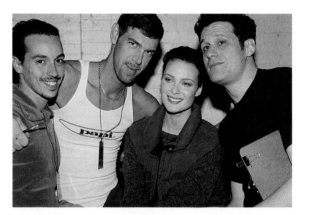

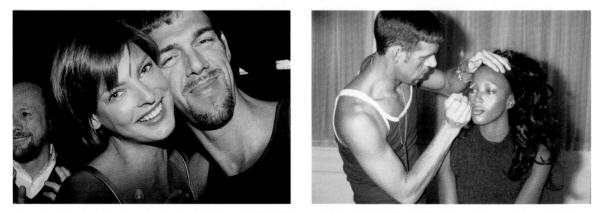

Above: Backstage buddies. Clockwise from top left: Kevyn with Todd Oldham and Kate; hairstylist Orlando Pita, Shalom Harlow, and Isaac Mizrahi; Naomi (Naomi photo: © Mitchell Gerber/CORBIS); and Linda.

were ready to face the barrage of photographers, or whatever it was you were facing that day."

"The designers obviously loved his makeup, but secondly, they thought the energy that he brought was great," explains makeup artist Charlie Green, who often assisted Kevyn at shows. "Backstage was a lot more of a party atmosphere then. Everybody knew each other—the caterers, the hairdressers, the security guards. There was champagne everywhere, so I'd always take two bottles and put them in Kevyn's kit. I'd say, 'Kevyn, be careful when you open your bag when you get home,' with a little wink and a nod. We certainly had our fun."

The season's hottest ticket was to the Perry Ellis show. The designer had died of AIDS in 1986, and the young, brash Marc Jacobs had been given the task of reviving the house. Jacobs shocked the fashion community by sending out a high-fashion version of grunge; Kevyn did minimal makeup to match. "You couldn't put on a lot of makeup if you were wearing these clothes, but I didn't want the girls to look like uncooked potato heads," Kevyn told former *Bazaar* editor Annemarie Iverson backstage.

The controversial collection eventually cost Jacobs his job. In retrospect, though, Jacobs's upscale take on street style was visionary. Change was afoot in the industry, and the supermodel phenomenon that *Time* had spotlighted only a year earlier was on the way out; a more laid-back approach to life, luxury, fashion, and even makeup was moving in. Just as this was happening, Kevyn got a call that would set a new direction for him as well. Janet Jackson wanted

him to do the makeup for the cover of her new album, *Janet.* "I had seen his portfolio and absolutely fell in love with his work," she says.

Patrick Demarchelier was the photographer, and the shoot took place in Miami. Jackson loved the soft, sexy look that Kevyn created for her, and, just as important, she adored Kevyn. She worked exclusively with him over the next several years for videos, photo shoots, talk shows, award shows, and personal appearances. Kevyn had worked with huge stars in the past, but this was the first time he had seriously teamed up with such a young, influential celebrity. She was his entrée to the white-hot epicenter of pop culture. Kevyn would rock this world, just as he had the fashion industry.

During the Janet Jackson whirlwind, Kevyn got a second chance to connect with Barbra Streisand during a *Vogue* shoot with Steven Meisel in the summer of '93. This go-round was a completely different experience. "The stories he told about seeing me when he was young and how it influenced his life were very affecting," says Streisand. "What a darling guy. His persona, his kindness, his good heart just seeped out through his pores."

The two kept in touch after the shoot, exchanging birthday cards and notes during the holidays. To this day, Streisand still uses a concealer that Kevyn sent her from Japan. "It's the perfect color for my skin," she says. "I'll be using it 'til the last drop. I think of him every day as I put it on."

The product was probably a prototype for Inoui, the prestige cosmetics line that Kevyn had been

ISSUE 665 · SEPTEMBER 16, 1993 · $2.95 · CAN $3.50 · UK £3.00

Rolling Stone

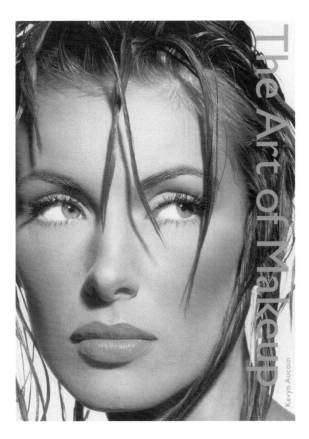

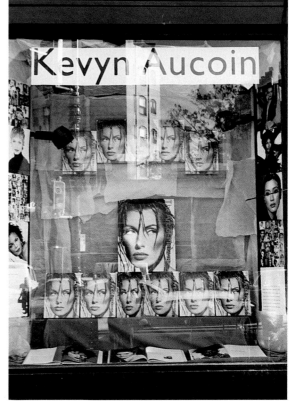

hired to revamp for Shiseido, the Asian beauty powerhouse. Kevyn developed all the products and directed the gorgeous ad campaigns, shot by Avedon and Meisel and featuring his favorite models, such as Kristen McMenamy, Jenny Shimizu, and Jaime Rishar. Japanese beauty fans carried on as if he were a rock star when he made department-store appearances in Tokyo.

In 1994, Kevyn was in the midst of working on his first book, *The Art of Makeup,* which had been the brainchild of Donald Reuter, his boyfriend. "Kevyn's portfolio was the inspiration," says Donald, who had been an assistant designer at Geoffrey

Beene. "Just flipping through it was such a joy. I remember thinking, 'My God, look at these celebrities, these models. What a great book this would be." A number of literary agents turned it down, but with the help of book producer Nicholas Callaway, *The Art of Makeup* eventually found a home at Harper-Collins. In the midst of the production process, Kevyn and Donald broke up, but they kept their professional relationship intact. Donald would go on to be the creative director of Kevyn's next two books.

The Art of Makeup, a combination of beauty advice, autobiography, and fabulous pictures, featured every celebrity, model, and photographer Kevyn had

Above: Kevyn's first book, *The Art of Makeup*, and a bookstore display.
Opposite, top: Kevyn and Milla Jovovich behind the scenes from an Inoui ad campaign shoot (photo by Eric Sakas).
Opposite, bottom: Kevyn and boyfriend Eric Sakas.

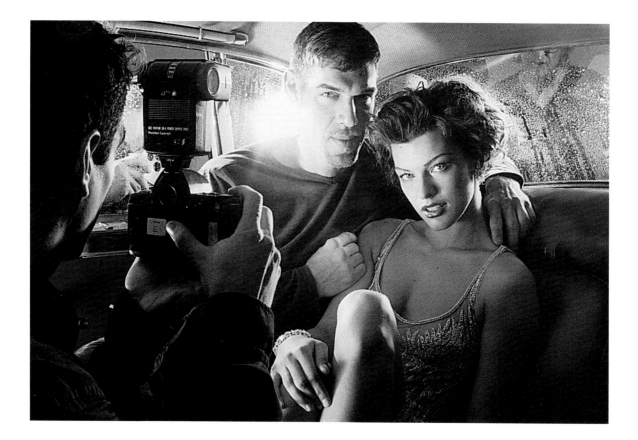

worked with up to that point. No makeup artist had produced anything remotely similar to it, for a simple reason: only Kevyn had that breadth of work.

Kevyn dedicated the book to his parents and the memory of his cousin Jay.

Everyone who saw *The Art of Makeup* was impressed. "I remember when the first article came out," says Marcy Engelman, Kevyn's close friend and publicist. "It was by Dana Wood in *W* magazine. I got the issue on the newsstand at ten o'clock at night and rushed to Kevyn's house in a taxi. We were both so excited. Kevyn sat there and read it over and over."

On November 2, Linda Wells and Sandy

Golinkin, the editor and publisher of *Allure,* respectively, threw a huge party at the Paula Cooper Gallery in SoHo to celebrate the publication. "Only in New York would you see a street blocked off for the launch of a makeup book," reported Jeanne Beker on Fashion Television. "But when you think of the makeup artist who came up with the book, Kevyn Aucoin, you kind of understand why."

The entrance was packed with guests and photographers when Kevyn arrived with Janet Jackson and his new boyfriend, Eric Sakas. "Kevyn, this is insanity of the highest order!" yelled Beker over the noise. "And you're the man of the moment."

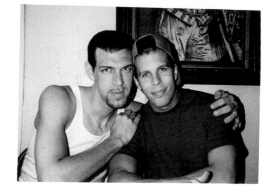

1995–1998

CHAPTER SIX

THE DREAM YEARS

"I don't want to be tolerated. I want to be celebrated."

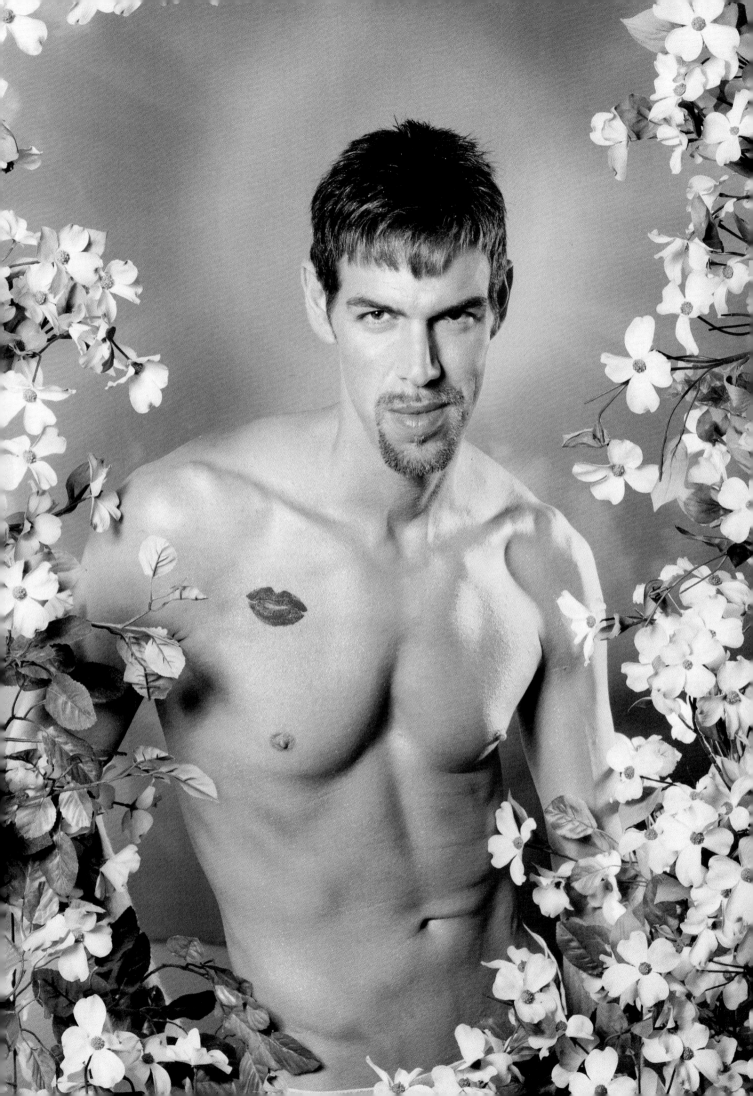

Preceding spread: Portrait of Kevyn from the cover of *Icon* magazine, by Eric Sakas.

Opposite: Kevyn's datebook entry from the CFDA Awards, with picture of Kevyn and his date for the night, supermodel Nadja Auermann.

Kevyn paced backstage at Lincoln Center as Janet Jackson's music burst from the sound system. The occasion was the annual CFDA Awards, the Oscars of fashion, and the Council of Fashion Designers of America was about to present Kevyn with a special award for his contributions to the industry. (He was, and would be to date, the only makeup artist ever honored by the organization.) The luminaries packed into the room—Donatella Versace, Karl Lagerfeld, Donna Karan, even Princess Diana, whom he had been introduced to earlier in the evening—watched as the most fierce and fabulous images Kevyn ever worked on flew across the video screen.

Suddenly, Roseanne Arnold appeared on the screen, lounging in bed, wearing a pink boa and dramatic makeup. "What I wouldn't pay to have Kevyn with me twenty-four hours a day to keep me looking and feeling this fantastic," she said. Just then, a hand reached over and powdered her face. The camera panned back to reveal Kevyn, half-asleep next to her, as the audience laughed hysterically. "Because I couldn't be there tonight, I'm sending my gorgeous German counterpart, Nadja Auermann," she said. "Take it away, Nadj."

With that, the Valkyrian supermodel strode across the stage and introduced Kevyn. Dressed in a black suit custom-made by Richard Tyler, he walked to the podium and started talking, his voice soft and nervous. He thanked the CFDA, the editors, designers, hairdressers, and photographers he had worked with, his parents, his new boyfriend Eric Sakas, and his dearest friends Jed Root, Donald Reuter, Marcy Engelman, and Linda Wells.

"I found it so hard to put into words exactly how I feel about receiving this incredible honor. You'll have to forgive me for being overly sentimental, for there's still a big part of me that can't believe that I made it out of Louisiana, that I live in New York, and that I'm here right now. I'm going to throw up! I'm sorry. Sorry.

"It seems like yesterday I was in my bedroom in Lafayette with my cousin Jay poring over fashion magazines and listening to Barbra Streisand records and fantasizing about our escape from the homophobic South. We found a temporary escape in the world of fashion and beauty, where all the models looked so happy, or at least interesting. Jay and I, like so many gay kids in America, were looking for a place where we could be free. Free, that is, to do any kind of hair or makeup styles we wanted. Or at least a place free from flying rocks, bottles, and shotgun shells. That's how we knew if our outfits were a hit.

"Anyway, Jay decided to stay in Louisiana, and I decided to move to New York City. Moving here was exciting and so different, except, of course, for the flying rocks, bottles, and shotgun shells. But at least they let boys do makeup here without having to see a state-appointed psychiatrist. After a lucky break, I began to work, and as I continued to work, I

kevyn aucoin: a beautiful life

CFDA AWARDS — TONIGHT I
WAS GIVEN a SPECIAL AWARD
FOR EXCELLENCE IN MAKE-UP
ARTISTRY — ROSEANNE made
a SPEECH ON VIDEO AND
NADYA Auerman PRESENTED
MY MOM & DAD & ERIC WERE
ALL THERE — IT WAS THE BEST
NIGHT OF MY LIFE — I'VE
DONE ALL I NEED TO DO — THE
REST IS EXTRA —

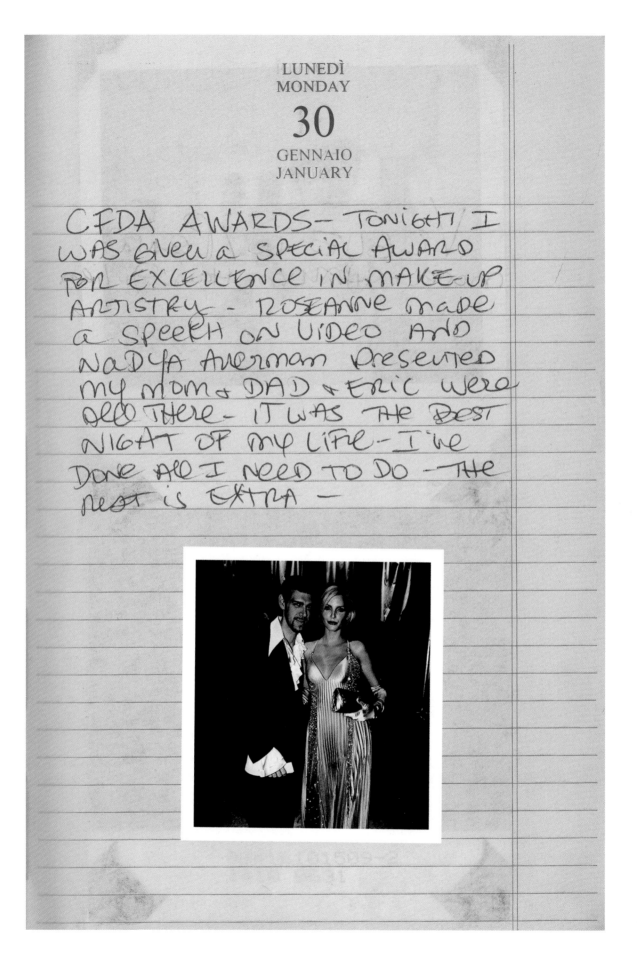

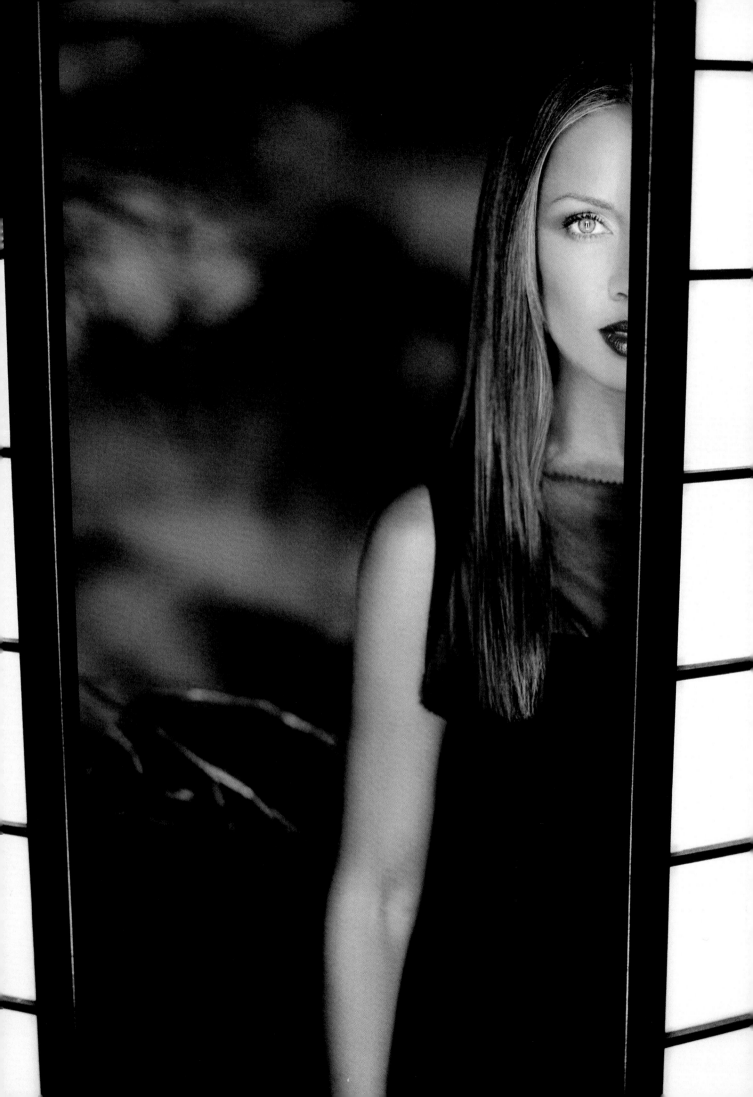

became more and more aware of how lucky I was as the phone calls from my cousin became more and more distressing. It seems that the life of an extremely effeminate, openly gay hairdresser in Lake Charles, Louisiana, was as scary as it sounds.

"After several attempts to get him to New York, Jay finally came. It was everything he'd dreamed it would be and more. It was during this time that he told me how proud he was of me, how tired he was of fighting, and that he had AIDS. A few months later, Jay died. It was only later that I realized this was the only way Jay felt he could escape. I know that to some people, winning an award for doing makeup may seem silly, but you see, in the context of my life, it means that I not only survived my past, but that I somehow succeeded. Thank you all very, very much for this honor."

The crowd broke into applause, and Kevyn left the stage. He rarely wrote personal notes in his datebook, but when he got home, he scribbled the following: "It was the best night of my life. I've done all I need to do. The rest is extra."

If Kevyn had a crystal ball, he would have realized how much was yet to come. At this point in his career, he hadn't worked on a single star for the Academy Awards, he hadn't published the book that hit number one on the *New York Times* bestseller list, nor had he launched his makeup line or his *Allure* column. He hadn't even met the women who would become such an integral part of his personal and professional life: Gwyneth Paltrow, Julia Roberts, Sharon Stone, Winona Ryder, Tori Amos, Courtney Love, Jewel, and Cher. Over the next few years, he would befriend all of them and become their makeup artist of choice.

Despite the fashion world accolades, the music industry was becoming more and more important to Kevyn's career. Each week he fielded additional requests to work on album covers and videos. He worked frequently with Vanessa Williams, who eventually hired him to do the photography *and* makeup for two of her album covers. Kevyn had been interested in photography since he was a child, so it was only natural that after years of watching the best in the business, he would finally get behind the camera. "He was a brilliant photographer," says Williams. "He knew exactly what he wanted to do, he was very relaxed, and lots of fun. He hired the stylist, the set decorators, and the lighting team and the pictures came out beautifully."

Around this time, Kevyn had begun working with Tori Amos, the flame-haired singer-songwriter who

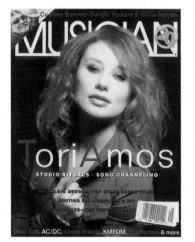

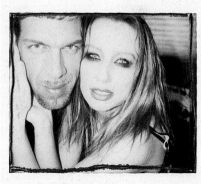

Opposite: Vanessa Williams by Kevyn from the photo shoot for her *Greatest Hits* album.
Right: Kevyn and Tori Amos.

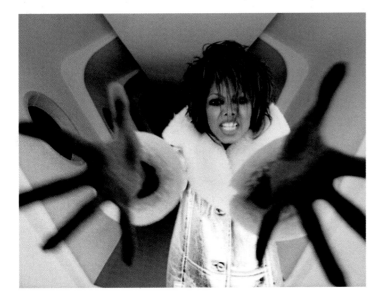

became one of his closest confidantes. Her emotionally charged lyrics and willingness to play with her appearance from project to project instantly attracted Kevyn. "He made me realize you don't have to feel like you're stepping into someone else's shoes when you change your look," says Amos, who later asked Kevyn to be the godfather to her firstborn child, Natashya. "He would say, 'Who are you really? Maybe that changes, and you have to allow that to change.' "

His most intense video of 1995 was Janet and Michael Jackson's space-age duet, "Scream," which involved a grueling eight-day shoot with director Mark Romanek and cost $7 million to produce. That year, Janet Jackson introduced Kevyn to her new sister-in-law, Lisa Marie Presley. He did her makeup for the *Primetime* interview with Michael Jackson, during which Diane Sawyer asked her to explain her marriage to the King of Pop.

Julia Roberts was already a big star when she and Kevyn worked together for the first time in 1995, on shoots with Herb Ritts and Peter Lindbergh. Gwyneth Paltrow, on the other hand, was better known for dating Brad Pitt than for

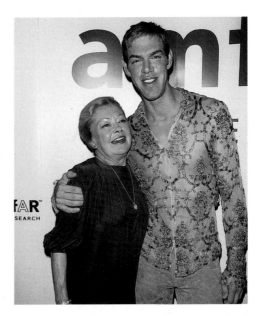

Top: Janet from the *Scream* video by Mark Romanek.
Right: Kevyn and Dr. Mathilde Krim at an AmFAR event.
Opposite: Lisa Marie Presley by Kevyn.

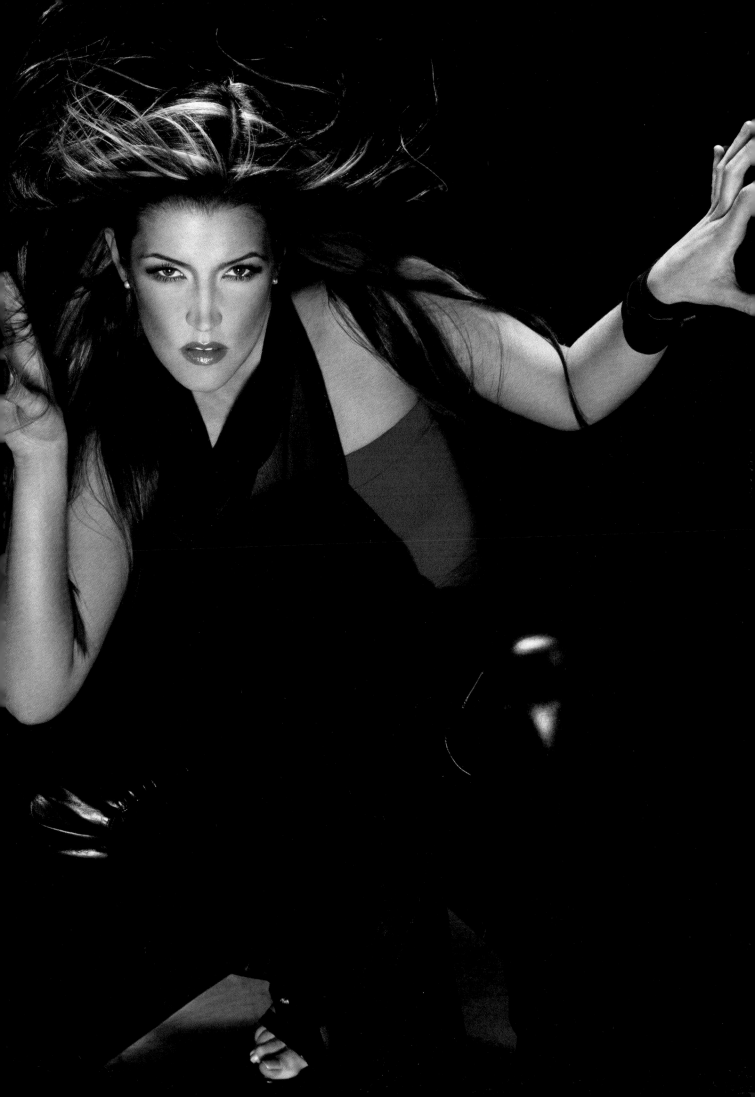

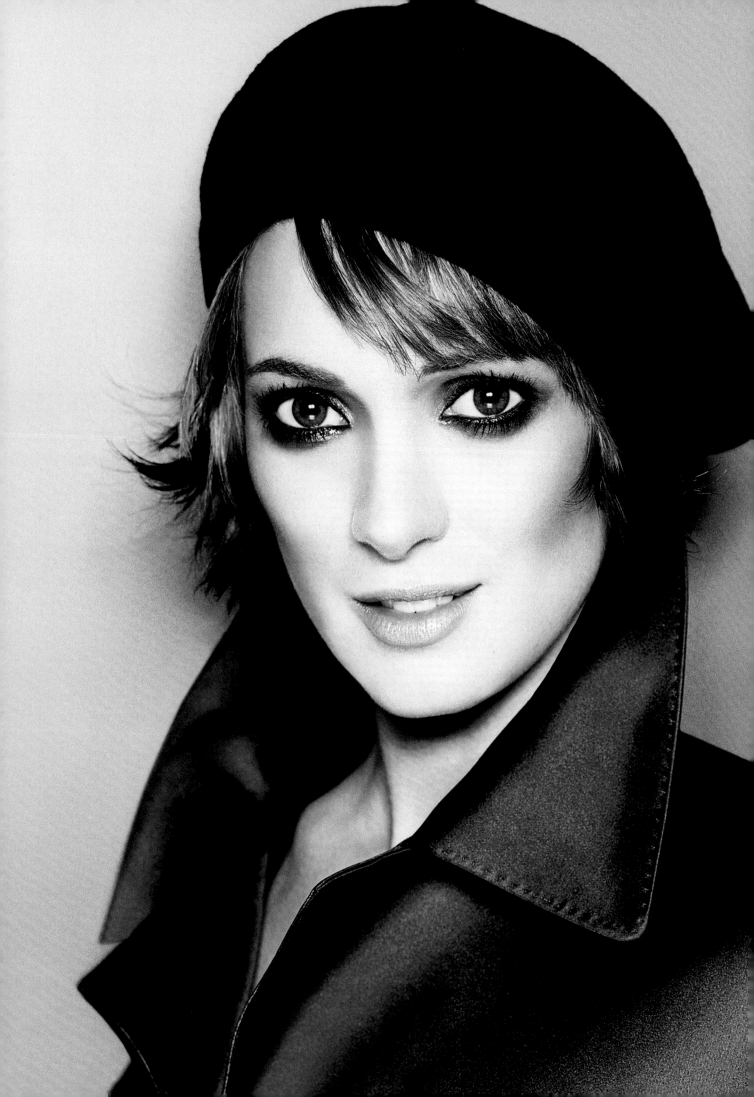

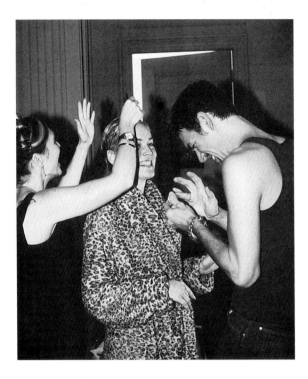

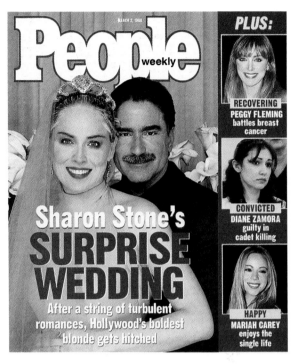

her acting career when she and Kevyn met. That was set to change with the release of *Emma,* an adaptation of the Jane Austen classic in which Paltrow played the title role.

In September 1996, Kevyn did Sharon Stone's makeup for the MTV Awards. Her beauty and her brains blew him away, but he especially admired her commitment to fighting AIDS. Kevyn offered to do her makeup for free any time she appeared on behalf of the American Foundation for AIDS Research

(AmFAR). "Let me ask you, who gives anything away for free?" says Stone. Kevyn did her makeup a few years later for her surprise Valentine's Day wedding to newspaper executive Phil Bronstein. Since it also was Kevyn's thirty-sixth birthday, Stone had a cake brought out for him before the wedding cake.

Kevyn also met Winona Ryder in September 1996. Her expressive face and big, soulful eyes were the ideal canvas for his makeup. "She has just about the most perfect face I've ever seen—like a porcelain

Opposite: Winona Ryder by Patrick Demarchelier for *Harper's Bazaar*. Above: Kevyn with Sharon Stone on her wedding day. Below: Kevyn and Winona.

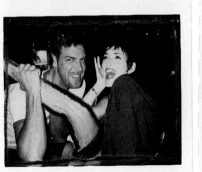

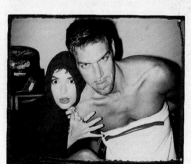

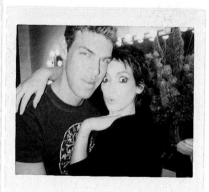

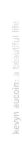

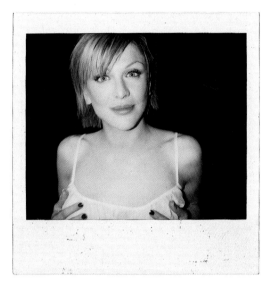

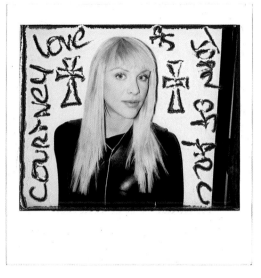

doll," rhapsodized Kevyn in *Allure.* A deep friendship developed between the two, and Kevyn and Ryder spent hours just hanging out at home, watching their favorite TV shows, movies, and documentaries.

Kevyn and the mercurial Courtney Love bonded at a *Vogue* shoot with Steven Meisel. Having temporarily traded in her guitar for an acting career, the alt-rock goddess was promoting her first major film, *The People vs. Larry Flynt.* Kevyn loved that she was political, confrontational, and as talkative as he was. He later did her makeup for a *Bazaar*

cover, the Golden Globes, and the Oscars. People were amazed at the transformation.

Kevyn's next big project was his new book, *Making Faces,* which focused on his beauty advice and celebrity transformations. Most important, it marked the emergence of Kevyn as a photographer in his own right, as more than half the work in the book was his. The first model he shot was one of his favorites, Chandra North. "Kevyn was very confident behind the camera," she says. "He'd give you lots of direction. We did some funny pictures

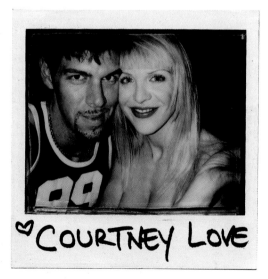

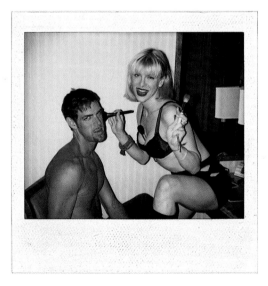

Above: Kevyn and Courtney Love. Opposite: Courtney by Steven Meisel © 1997 *Vogue*. Courtesy of Condé Nast Publications Inc.

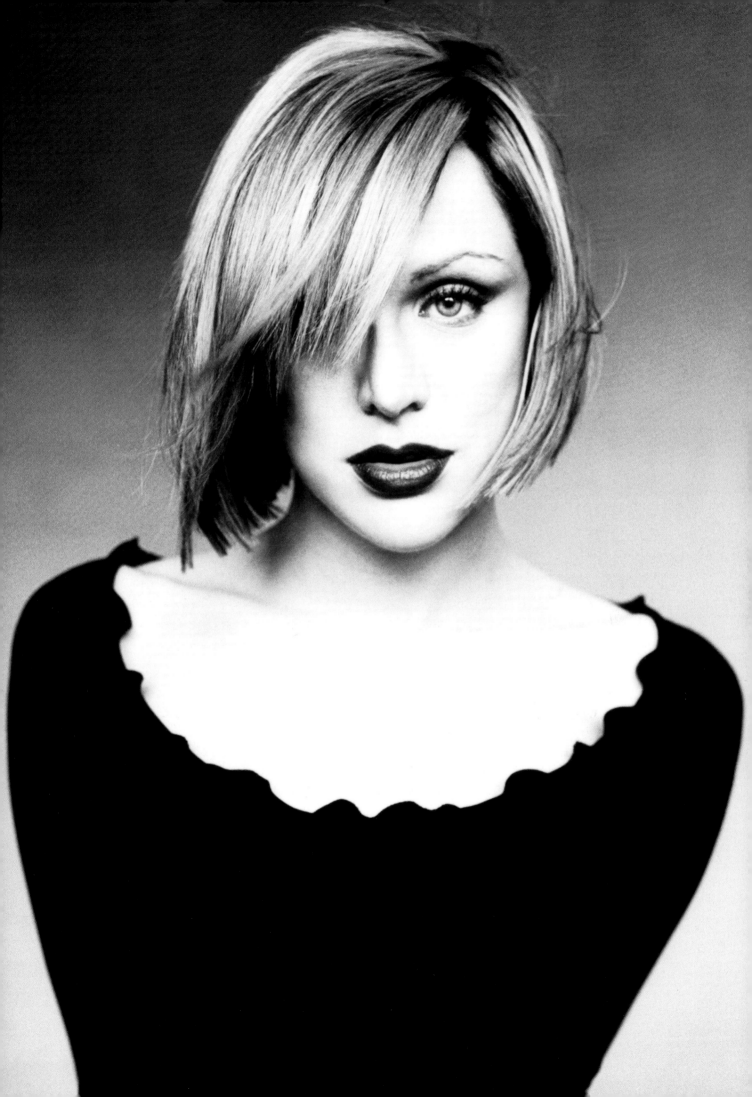

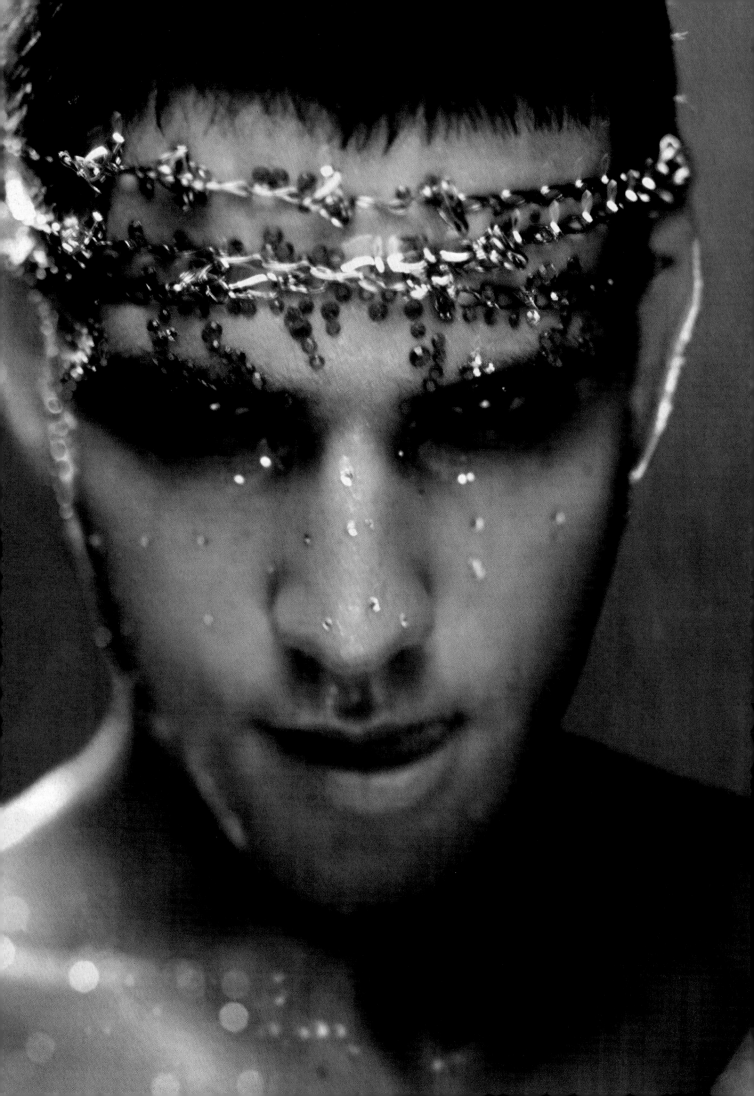

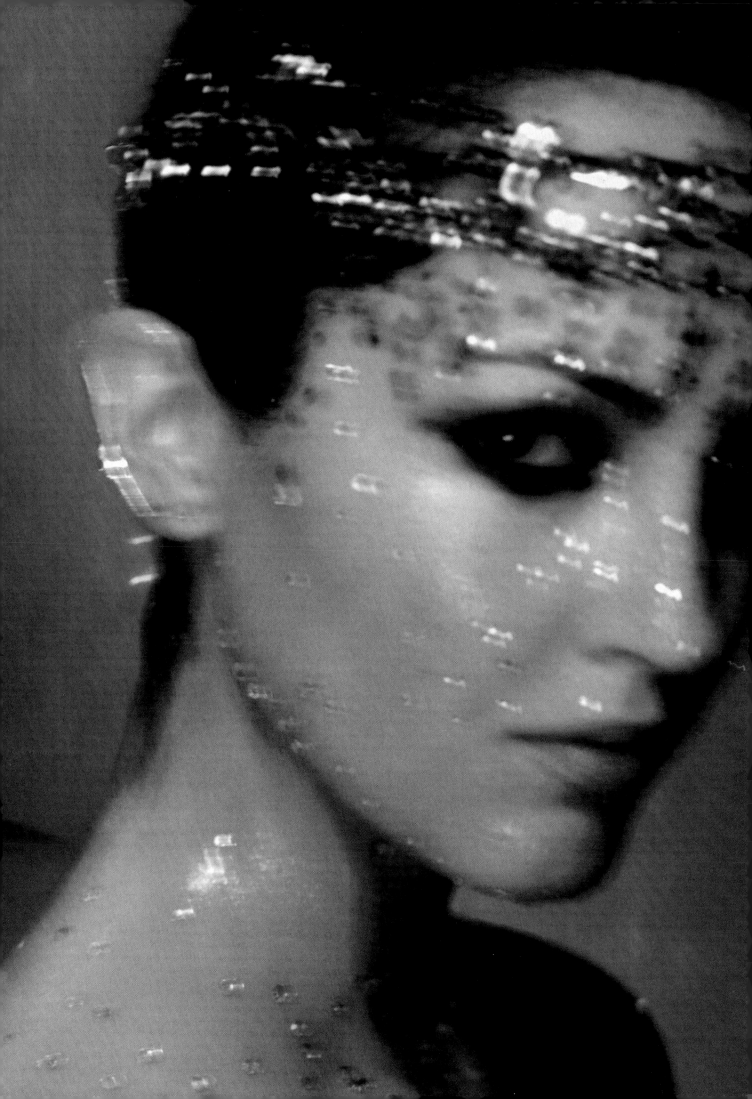

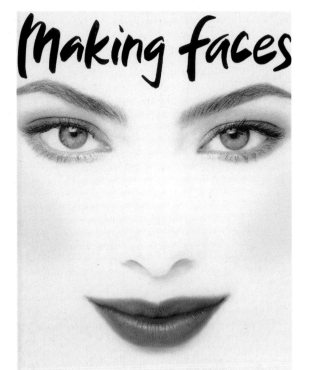

Making faces

KEVYN AUCOIN

Preceding spread: Rubin Singer and Chandra North
by Kevyn for *Flaunt* magazine.
Left: The cover of *Making Faces*.
Below: The book's cover girl, Shalom.
Opposite: Chandra by Kevyn for *Spur* magazine.

where he said, 'I want you to look like somebody is about to take your purse!' It was the emotion he was after. With his beauty pictures, getting the right expression in the eyes was so important."

The first famous face he morphed was Lisa Marie Presley into Marilyn Monroe. "Kevyn claimed that he saw Marilyn in my face the very first time he met me," says Presley. "I thought he was crazy."

Kevyn also turned the spotlight on his mother, Thelma, and his sisters Carla and Kim in *Making Faces.* After the book was published, all were approached for autographs. Someone even asked Thelma for hers in the parking lot of the local Wal-Mart. To Kevyn's fans, his family was as famous as the models and movie stars in the book.

Making Faces hit stores in fall 1997. It was selling moderately well when Kevyn made an appearance on *The Oprah Winfrey Show.* He transformed the talk-show host into Diana Ross and discussed some of the more dramatic makeovers in the book, such as Courtney Love as Jean Harlow and Demi Moore as Clara Bow. After the show aired, the book shot to number one. "I'm a high school dropout with a *New York Times* bestseller, so the irony of that is hilarious," said Kevyn.

During his book tour, he met hundreds of his fans, some of whom stood in line for hours just to talk to him; many burst into tears and told Kevyn he had changed their lives with his empowering message. At the start of each book signing, Kevyn told the store manager that he wasn't leaving until he had met every person in attendance. They all complied and sometimes had to leave the shop open an extra hour or two.

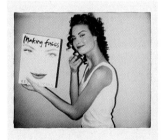

kevyn aucoin: a beautiful life

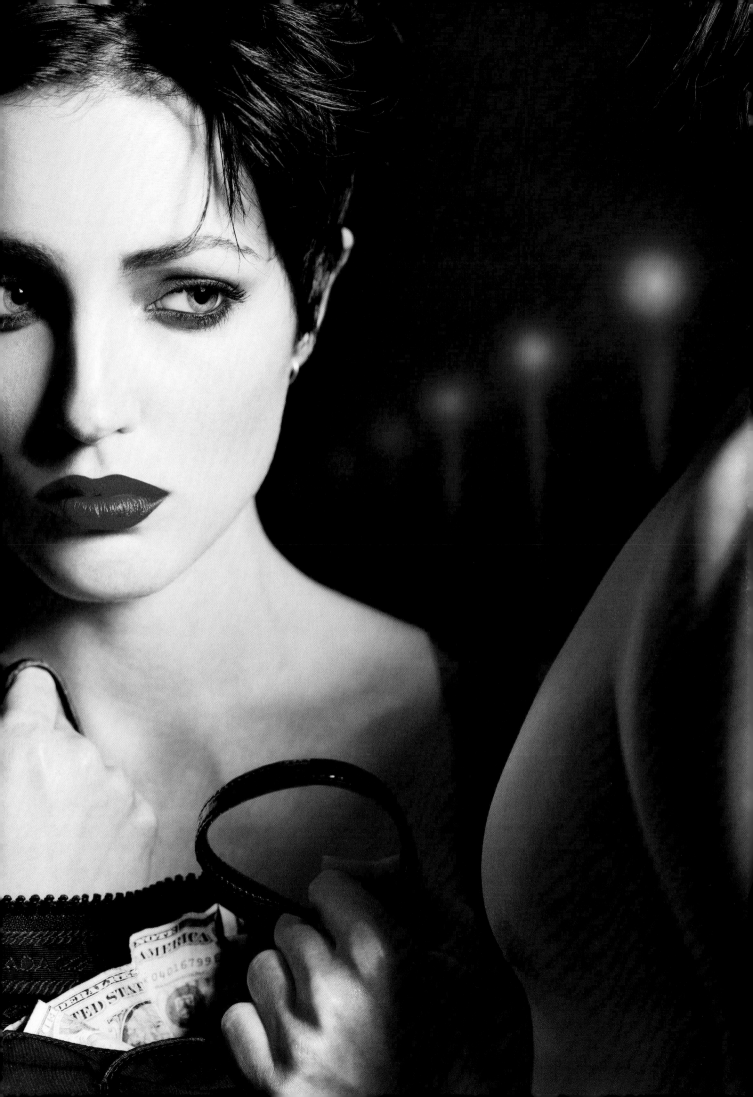

"HE WAS REALLY FUNNY. HE HAD A TREMENDOUSLY SICK SENSE OF HUMOR. I HAVE A VERY DARK, ACERBIC SENSE OF HUMOR, AND HE'S ONE OF THE FEW PEOPLE THAT YOU COULD GET AS DARK WITH AS YOU WANTED. NO JOKE WAS TOO DISGUSTING FOR HIM."

—JEWEL

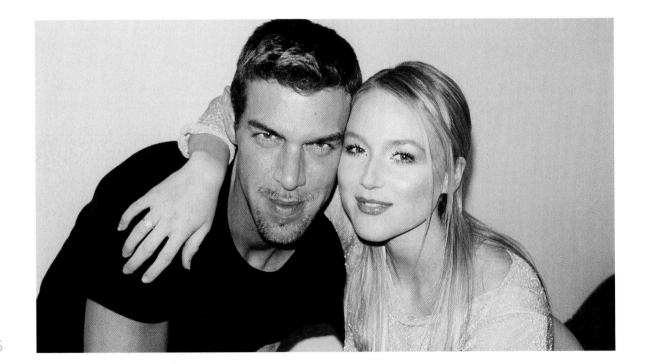

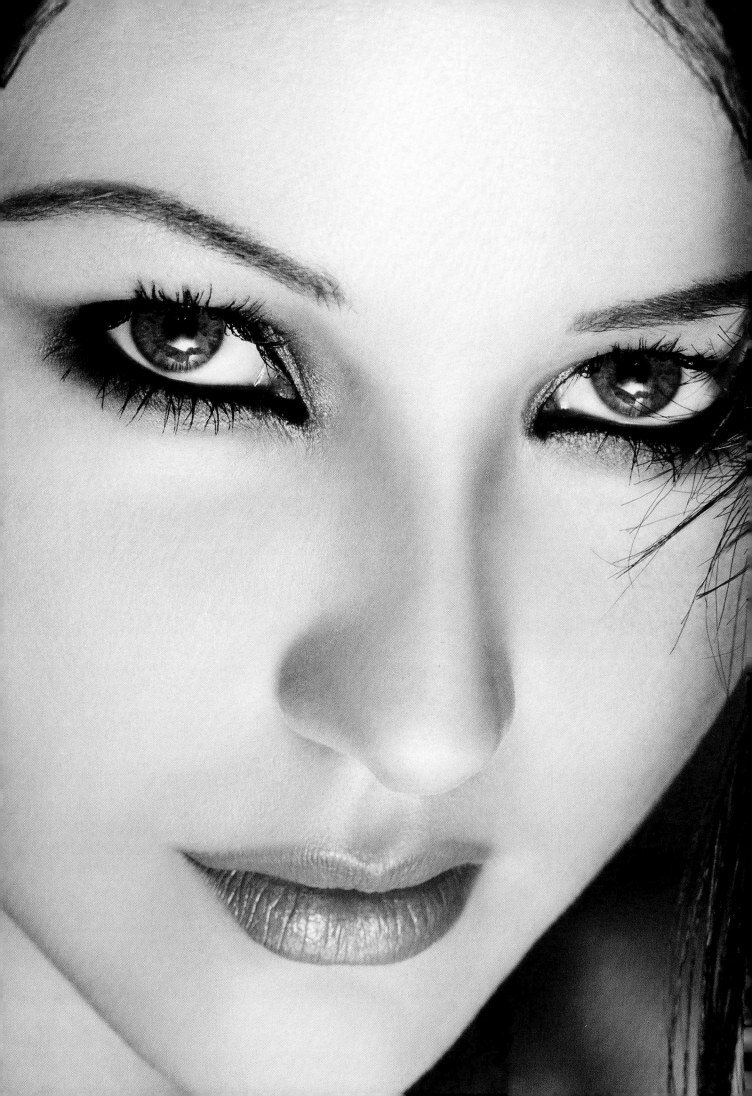

Even the celebrities who inspired the transformations loved the book. "When I first saw Isabella Rossellini as me, I thought, 'This guy is a genius,'" says Barbra Streisand. "Kevyn copied that picture from *Funny Girl* right down to the earrings. I never knew what happened to those earrings, and then one day I rented a boat in Mexico, and the captain says to me, 'My mother has your earrings from *Funny Girl.* You had a coat at that time, a fur coat, and you brought it in to be cleaned, and those earrings were in the pocket, and she kept them.' I said, 'Can you give them back? It's more than thirty years later and you know, *they're mine.*' They were fake, but I wanted them for sentimental reasons. He never sent them back. I think I told that story to Kevyn at one point because he actually re-created the earrings for the picture."

As 1998 dawned, Kevyn was becoming as cele-brated as his famous friends. *Cosmopolitan*'s "Last Gasp" column featured paparazzi photos of Kevyn with the likes of Liza Minnelli, Janet Jackson, and Paula Abdul. "Being worthy enough to wrangle an appointment with makeup artist to the stars Kevyn Aucoin is such a fashionable score that these fa-mous faces love to drag him out on the town to prove he did them up," read the article.

In a hilarious case of mistaken identity, some tabloids ran paparazzi photos of Kevyn with Cher, Cindy Crawford, and Elizabeth Hurley, in each case declaring Kevyn the star's new love interest.

American Photo magazine named Kevyn one of 1998's most important people in photography. "Most makeup artists are little-known craftsmen toiling away behind the scenes of the fashion busi-ness," it reported. "Kevyn Aucoin is a star." In the accompanying interview, Kevyn challenged the

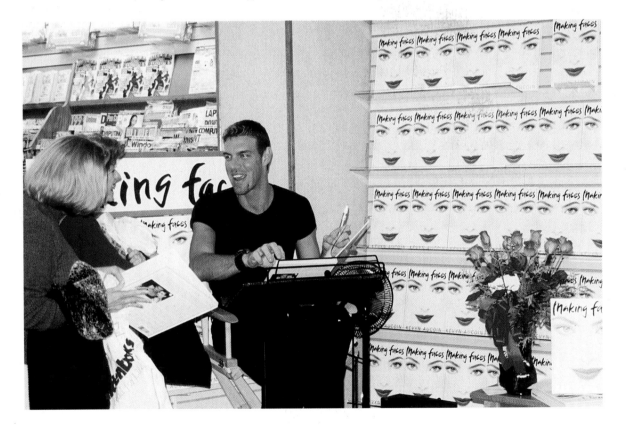

Above: Homecoming—Kevyn at the book signing for *Making Faces* in Lafayette, Louisiana.
Opposite: Chandra in drag by Kevyn. This was shot for *Making Faces* but rejected by the publisher.

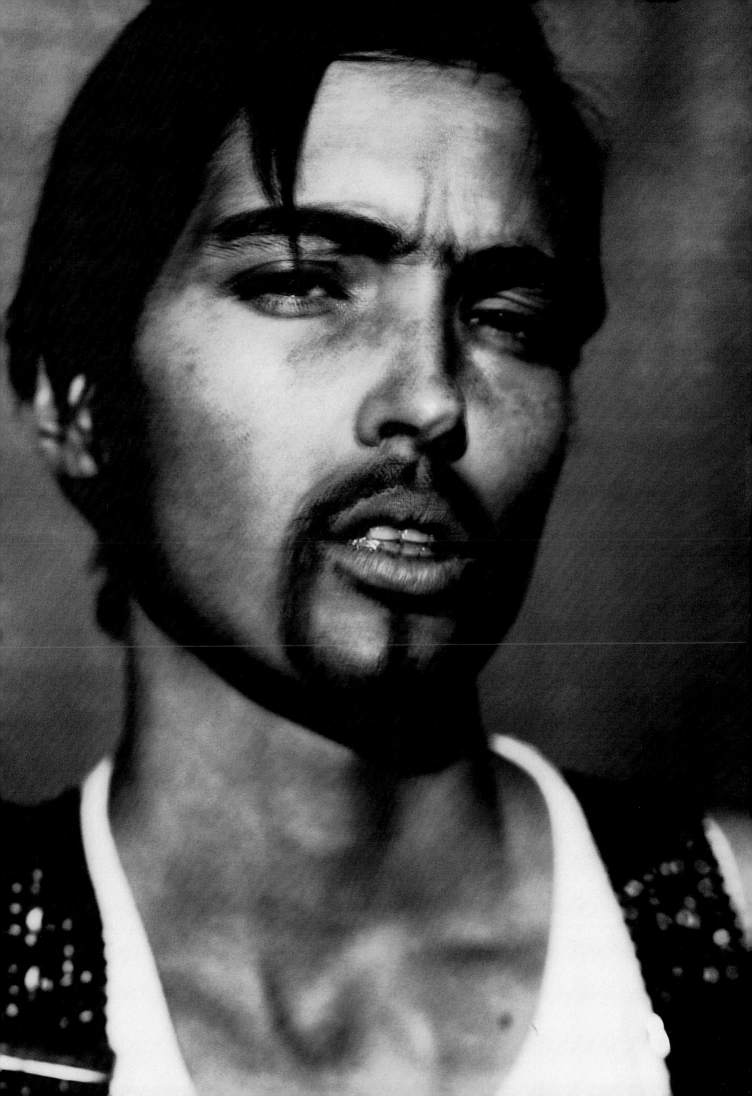

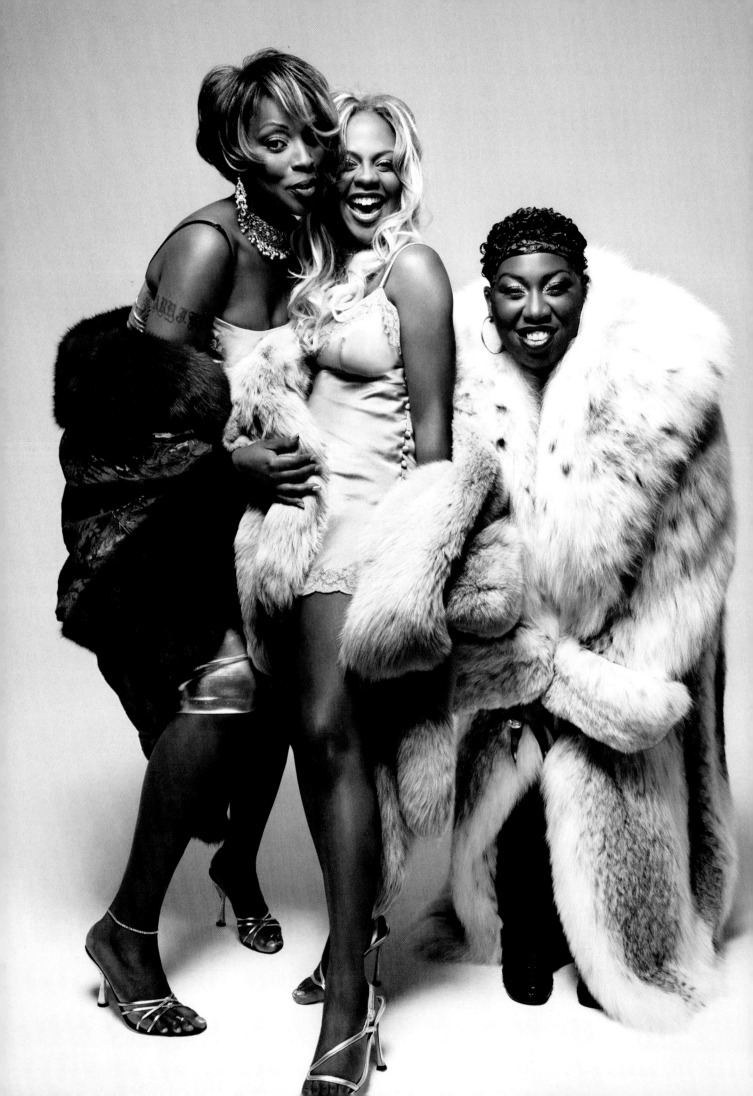

Left: Mary J. Blige, Lil' Kim, and Missy Elliot by Michael Thompson
for *Vogue* © Condé Nast Publications Inc.
Below: Behind the scenes. Right: Kevyn's collage.

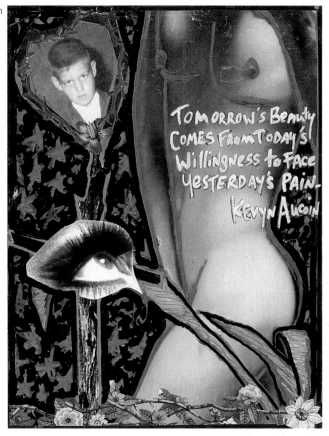

magazine that had championed him fifteen years earlier. "I'd like to see more black women on the cover of *Vogue*," he said. "We live in America, not Sweden."

Toward year's end, Kevyn was inducted into the *Allure* Hall of Fame alongside a few other beauty classics—Cindy Crawford, Chanel No. 5, and Retin-A. Another beauty industry honor came from Cosmetic Executive Women (C.E.W.). The organization recognized that Kevyn did more than make women look good; he influenced their purchases. Whenever he recommended a product, women ran to the store,

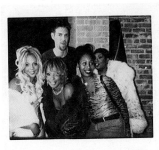

whether they were super-models on shoots or college kids reading

Allure. He was a hit maker and could help unknown brands become highly desirable commodities. "Other makeup artists talked about us, but nothing had the same impact as when Kevyn did," says Jami Morse Heidegger, whose family established Kiehl's, the cult grooming line that Kevyn helped popularize. "He talked from the heart and said what he believed in. He always wanted to share his secrets and help people look better and feel better."

Diane Sawyer presented Kevyn with his C.E.W. award. "Kevyn learned the greatest lesson I think you can learn in life, the one courageous lesson, which is how to use tears and suffering as a river to take you someplace, and where it took him was to a place full of light and love," she said.

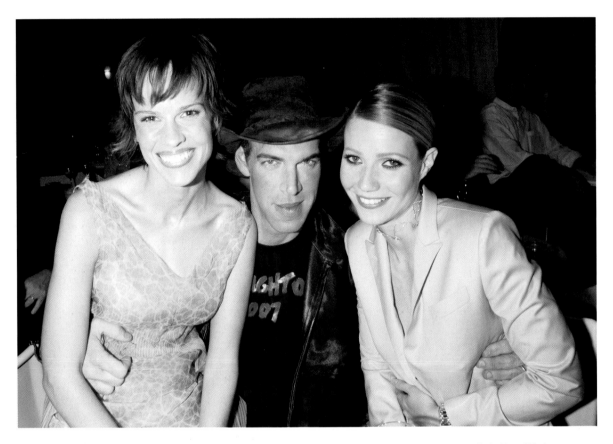

Kevyn and his Oscar winners: Hilary Swank and Gwyneth Paltrow at the 2001 *Vogue* VH-1 Fashion Awards. Photo: © Kevin Mazur/WireImage.com

KEVYN AND THE ACADEMY AWARDS

In March 1994, Janet Jackson called Kevyn and booked him for her Academy Awards appearance. Kevyn had never done anyone's makeup for the Oscars, but the ceremony was becoming a bigger fashion event with each passing year. In 1995, Oprah Winfrey was a presenter, wearing a chocolate brown gown by Dolce & Gabbana and makeup by Kevyn.

He worked with Nicole Kidman in 1996, when she made a splash in periwinkle Prada. The following year, he broke the rule about redheads and red lipstick and gave her a sexy scarlet pout to contrast with her chartreuse Dior gown. The look rocketed Nicole to the top of everyone's best-dressed list, but the big news of the night was his transformation of Courtney Love from grunge goddess to glamorous movie star. VH1 called it the makeover of the decade. "To be almost thirty when you find out that you're actually not the ugliest person in the world—he gave me that," says Love. "My manner changed, my posture changed. I didn't have to throw a bottle at anyone's head. I could be graceful, I could be gracious, and I could be nice."

Kevyn's biggest Oscar moment came in 1999. Gwyneth Paltrow had been nominated as Best Actress for her role in *Shakespeare in Love,* and she asked Kevyn and Orlando Pita, his good friend and top hairstylist, to help her get ready. They all met in Santa Monica at Shutters on the Beach, one of Paltrow's favorite hotels, along with her mother, Blythe Danner, and her best friend. Paltrow had decided

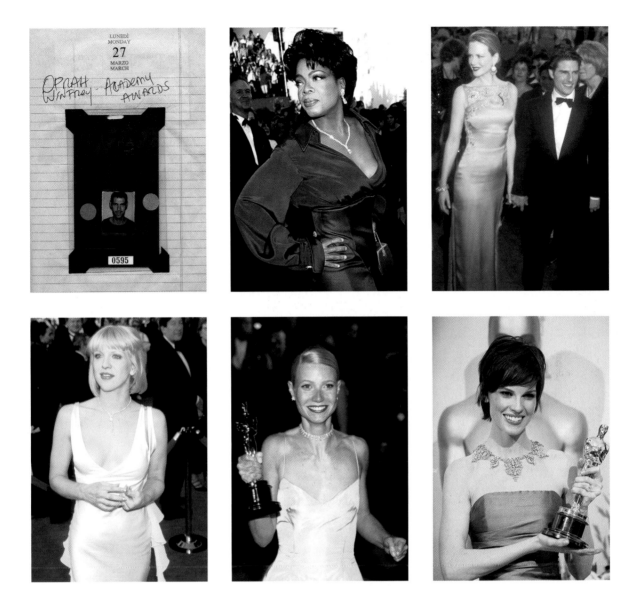

to wear a bubble-gum pink Ralph Lauren gown after deliberating between that and an icy blue Michael Kors dress. It took Kevyn and Orlando less than an hour to do the simple hair and makeup they devised for her. She hit the red carpet looking like a princess and was hailed as the new Grace Kelly. Kevyn was the least surprised person that night when Paltrow won in her category.

The next year, Kevyn worked with Hilary Swank, a little-known actress nominated for her role in the harrowing *Boys Don't Cry*. The production company for the indie film couldn't afford Kevyn's fee, but he

had been so impressed by the movie and by Swank that he offered to do her makeup for free. "Our budget was $1.6 million, so we didn't have a lot of money to do things with," says Swank. "Kevyn made me feel so calm that day. He put on some music and propped up some pillows so I could lay back. I don't have a lot of things on videotape, but I have that and I'm so glad. The whole experience with Kevyn was so amazing."

Kevyn proved to be a good luck charm two years in a row, as Swank, in a surprise win, took home the Oscar.

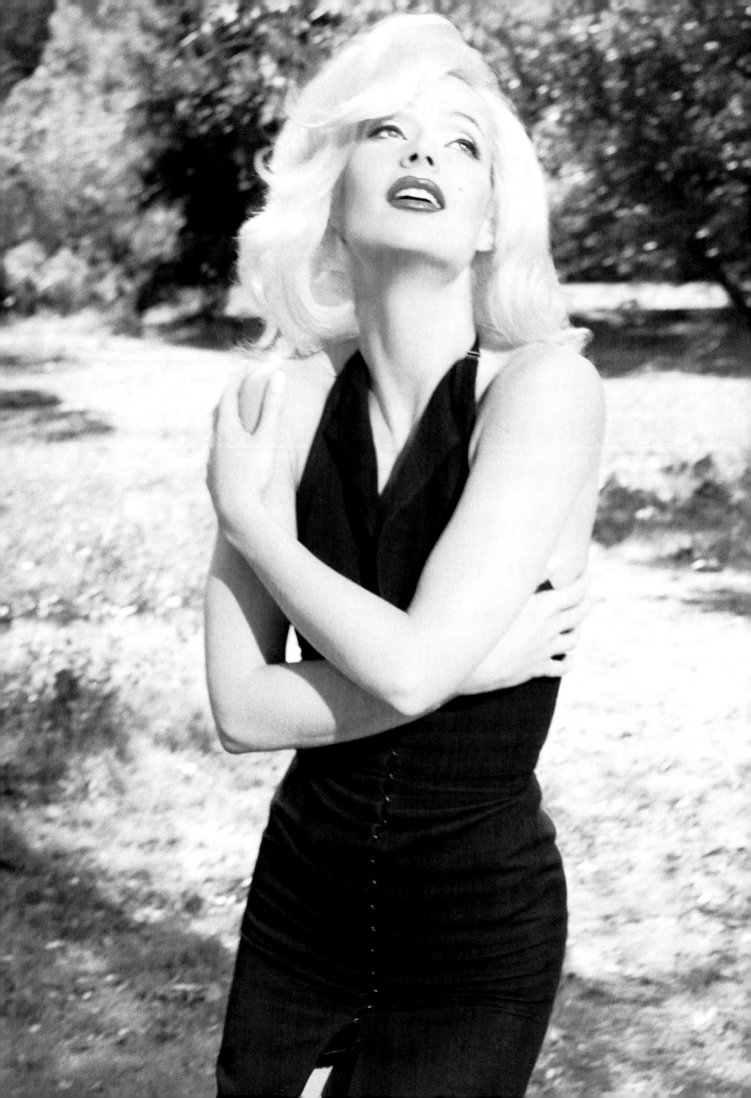

Opposite: Gwyneth as Marilyn Monroe by Herb Ritts. This picture is from the last shoot Gwyneth did with both Kevyn and Herb.

CHAPTER SEVEN

THE LEGEND YEARS
1999–2002

"Life is too short to spend it hoping that the perfectly arched eyebrow or hottest new lip shade can mask an ugly heart."

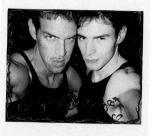

In January, Kevyn started dating Jeremy Antunes, an aspiring playwright from Rhode Island. "When our eyes first met a distinct feeling of déjà vu consumed us both," Kevyn would later write. He was so nervous about their first dinner that he dragged along his friend Gina Gershon, the actress best known for her role in the camp classic *Showgirls.* The relationship between Kevyn and Jeremy grew serious, and they started living together in Kevyn's duplex apartment in New York's Chelsea neighborhood.

One of the surprising facts about Kevyn's career at this point is how little he had worked with Madonna. They had so much in common: they were at the top of their fields, they loved transformations, they pushed buttons and boundaries, and they embraced sexual and racial diversity. Kevyn had done Madonna's makeup once, in 1997, for *Rolling Stone*'s Women of Rock issue, but throughout her career, Madonna mostly collaborated with two other great makeup artists, Francois Nars and Laura Mercier. In spring 1999, however, she asked Kevyn to work on the video for "Beautiful

Stranger," her single from the *Austin Powers* soundtrack. Next, they worked together on the video for "Power of Goodbye," a track from Madonna's *Ray of Light* album. Kevyn gave Madonna hauntingly beautiful makeup to go with her evocative lyrics.

Around the same time, Tommy Mottola, then the head of Sony Records, called about a new singer the label felt had major potential: Jennifer Lopez. Kevyn agreed to work with her, as he knew her from the set of Janet Jackson's "That's the Way Love Goes." (Lopez was a dancer in the video, and Kevyn did Jackson's makeup.) Kevyn and Oribe, the hairstylist, gave Lopez a sleek new look for the cover of her album, *On the 6,* and they worked on a twenty-four-hour, back-to-back video shoot for two of her singles, "If You Had My Love" and "No Me Ames," a duet with Marc Anthony. "We all took tons of vitamins; I drank gallons of Coca-Cola," wrote Kevyn in his new *Allure* column, "Kevyn's Notebook," which had launched that summer. "Jennifer's one of those chemical-free people. She's got so much natural drive, she doesn't need anything else."

Top: Kevyn and Jeremy Antunes.

Below: Kevyn and Madonna.

Opposite: Three icons, one photo: Courtney, Tina, and Madonna by Peggy Sirota © 1997 *Rolling Stone* LLC. All rights reserved. Reprinted by permission.

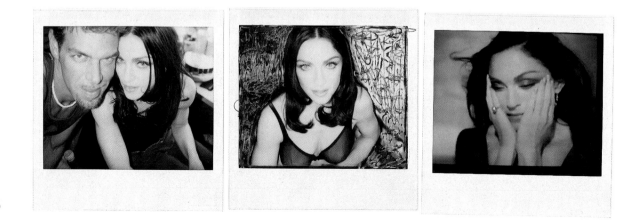

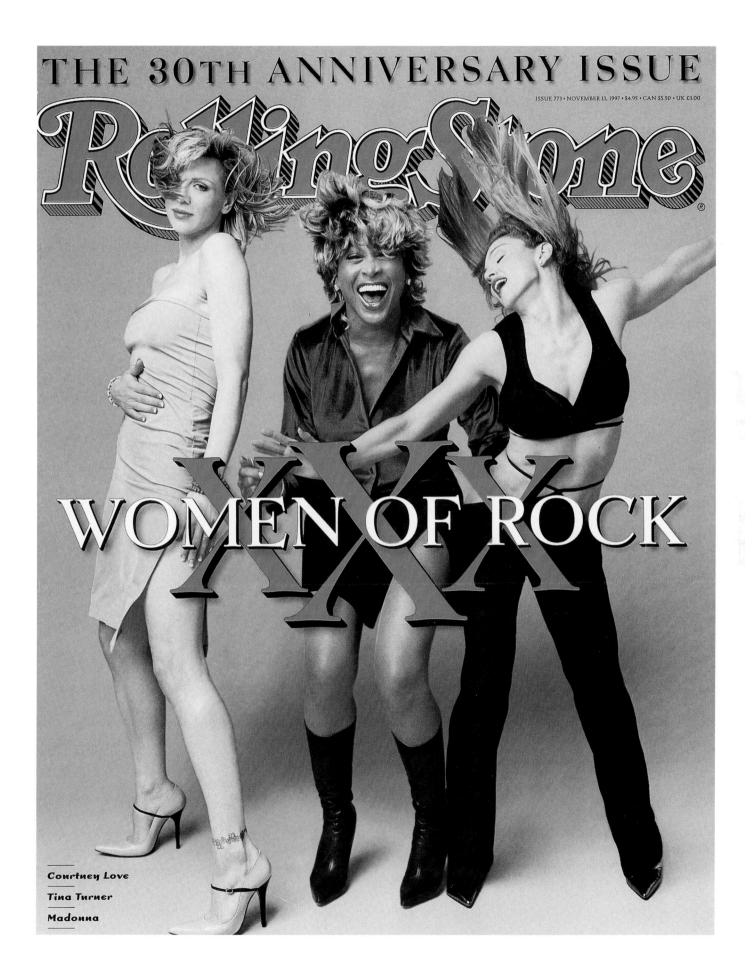

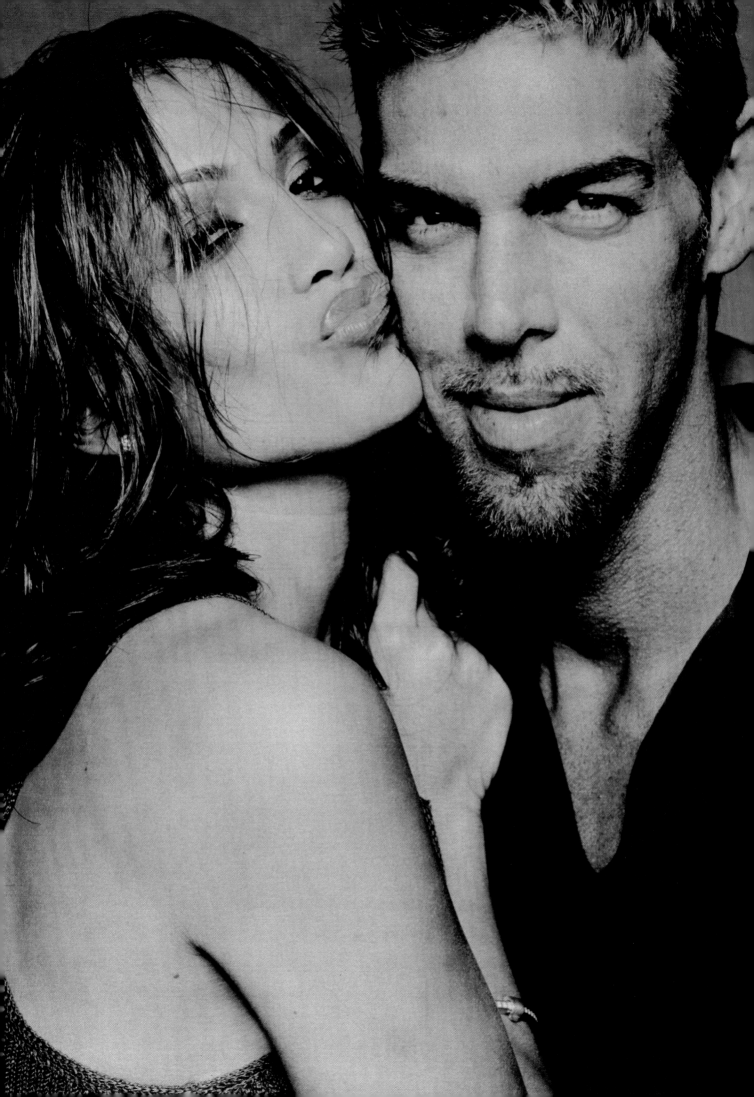

Kevyn and Oribe also teamed up to do "Waiting for Tonight," Lopez's video set at a millennium eve rave. Kevyn airbrushed her skin a deep bronze shade and glued hundreds of tiny crystals to her face so it would literally dance with light for the cameras. "That shoot was craziness," recalls Oribe. "Jennifer sat for four hours while Kevyn created that diamond face on her."

Over in cyberspace, meanwhile, the Internet beauty boom was under way. More than a dozen Web sites were set to launch, and several were courting Kevyn to come on board as a contributor or columnist. He accepted an offer from Beauty.com, the site founded by entrepreneur Roger Barnett, which Kevyn felt had the most promise. Venture capital money was flowing freely in those days, and according to industry sources, Kevyn was paid $1.2 million for a year's work. Additionally, he was given an ownership stake in the company.

Kevyn proved he was worth every penny during an *Oprah* appearance where he revealed his must-have items available on Beauty.com. The products sold out, and the site did more than a million dollars' worth of business in three days. (Kevyn later would part ways with Beauty.com when the site was acquired by Drugstore.com.)

Kevyn almost spent a big chunk of his Beauty.com salary in a single day. Among his many obsessions was Marilyn Monroe, so when he discovered that Christie's was auctioning her personal property—including her cosmetics—he picked up the phone and arranged for a personal viewing. Kevyn got to see everything from her "Happy Birthday, Mr. President" dress to her white baby grand piano (later bought by Mariah Carey), all the way down to her potholders.

On the day of the auction, Kevyn stayed behind, and Eric Sakas went in his place. Eric and Kevyn had broken up at this point, but Eric remained in his life as one of his best friends and his business partner. Kevyn was afraid that if someone recognized him, it would inflate the price of lot 310, Marilyn's traveling makeup case and its contents, which was estimated at $15,000. Even without Kevyn there, the price skyrocketed. "I was sitting on the phone with Kevyn, and he kept telling me to raise the bid," says Eric. "He thought that maybe the Beauty.com people would be willing to pay for it, but we dropped out at $150,000." Ripley's Believe It or Not bought Marilyn's makeup for $266,500.

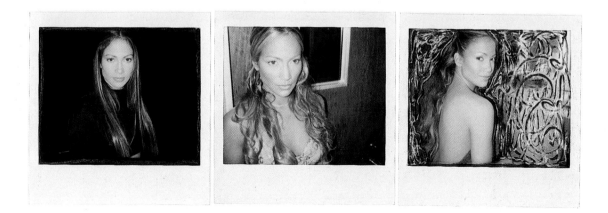

Opposite: Jennifer Lopez and Kevyn, by Kevyn. Above: Behind the scenes with Jennifer.

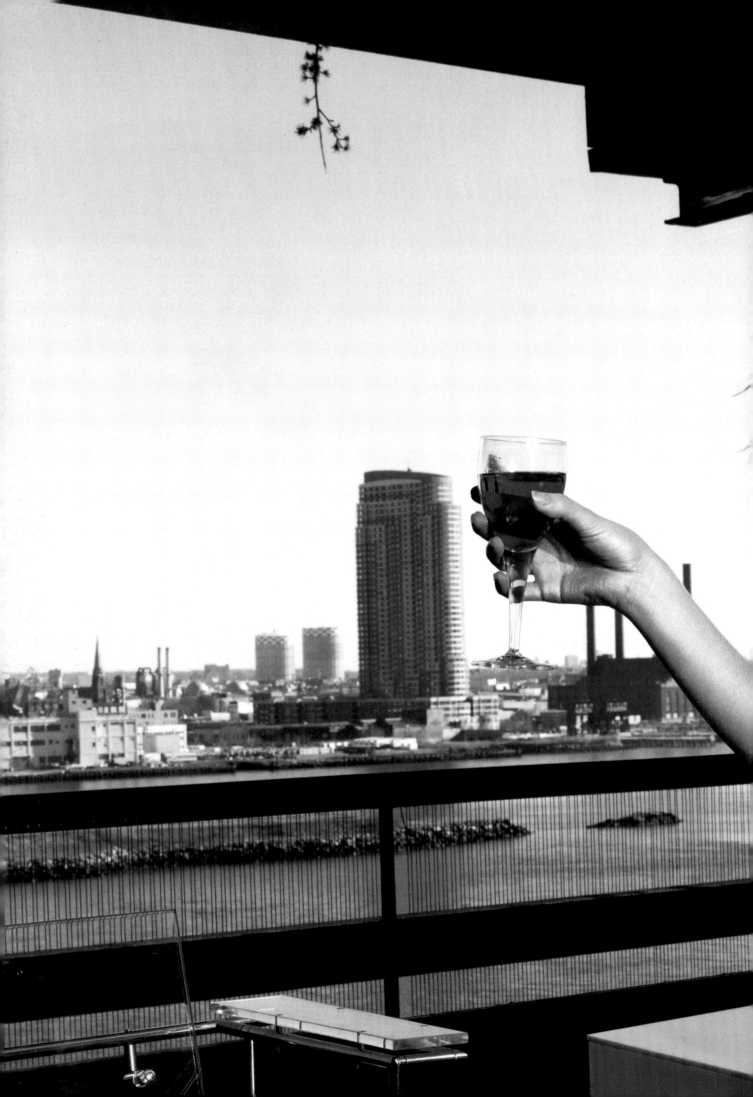

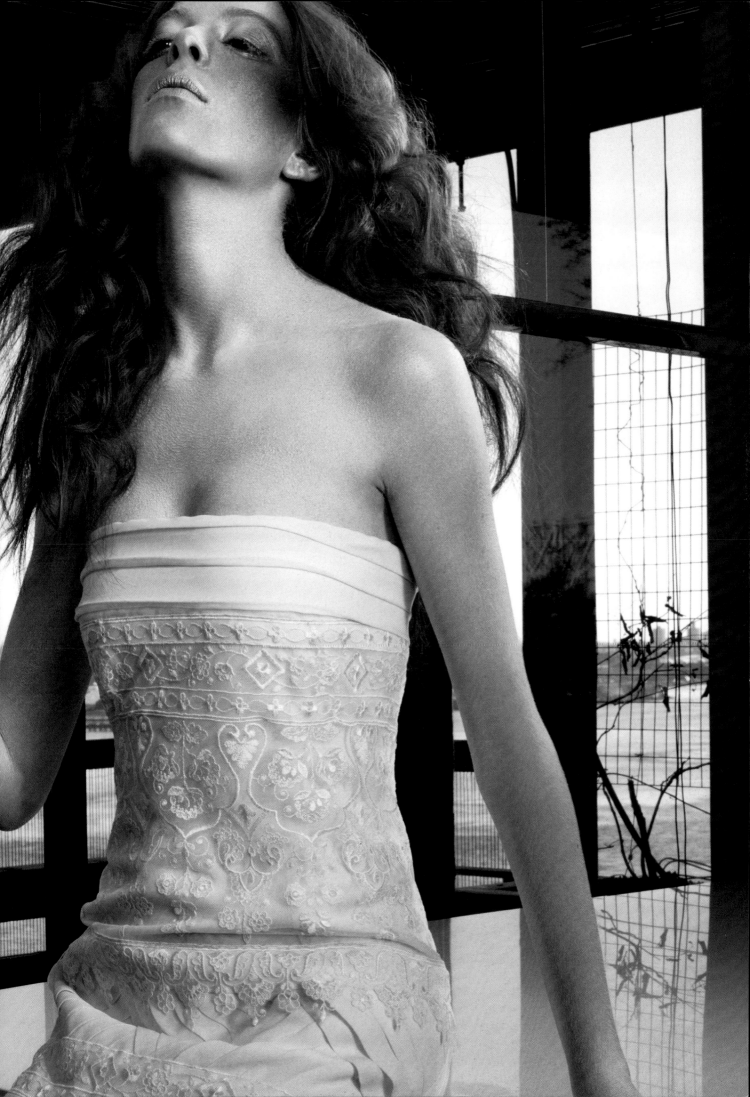

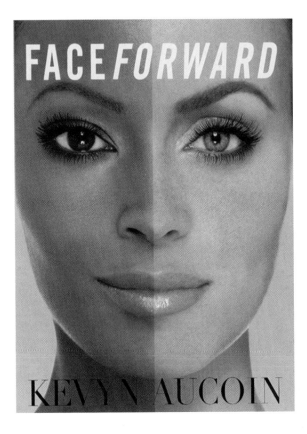

FACE*FORWARD*

KEVYN AUCOIN

At the time, Kevyn was laboring furiously to complete his third book, *Face Forward,* which featured even more of the celebrity transformations that were such a hit in his last book. Kevyn took almost every photo, and he and his team worked on back-to-back shoots to accommodate everyone's hectic schedule, including his own. It was like a celebrity assembly line. Gwyneth Paltrow would run in for an hour, followed by Julianne Moore, Celine Dion, and Mary J. Blige.

The transformations this time around were even more dramatic. When Gena Rowlands came in, she was floored by Kevyn's plans to turn her into Ava Gardner. "I thought he'd gone totally mad," recalls Rowlands. "I said, 'I know you're a genius, but there have to be some limits.' " Other highlights included

Martha Stewart as Veronica Lake, Alexandra von Furstenberg as Cher, and Hilary Swank as Raquel Welch. Kevyn was especially proud to include his transgendered friend Eveline Lange, whom he made up as Debbie Harry. *Face Forward* became another bestseller for Kevyn.

At the end of 1999, Kevyn finally got his high school diploma. The Hetrick-Martin Institute, which runs the Harvey Milk high school for gay teens in Greenwich Village, presented him with an honorary certificate. "Kevyn's passion and commitment to Hetrick-Martin was extraordinary," says board chairman Bari Mattes. "He made the young people feel so special each and every time he visited." Hetrick-Martin was one of Kevyn's favorite causes, and over the years he participated in career week, brought Liza Minnelli by to talk to the students, and donated dozens of copies of his books when they were published.

"Kevyn really believed in Hetrick-Martin," says Hilary Swank, who became the national spokesperson for the organization after portraying a gay teen in the movie *Boys Don't Cry.* "With his background and his childhood, it was something Kevyn wished he had when he was growing up."

"Today, many people do benefits, charities, everything is so public," says Donatella Versace, who got to know Kevyn after years of working together on fashion shows and shoots. "Kevyn did so much, and nobody knew."

Preceding spread: Steven Klein 1999 Italian *Vogue.* Courtesy of Condé Nast Publications Inc. Above: The cover of *Face Forward.* Right: Kevyn with a student from the Hetrick-Martin Institute; Kevyn's diploma. Opposite: Behind the scenes of Tina's Cleopatra shoot for *Face Forward* at the L'Ermitage Hotel in Beverly Hills.

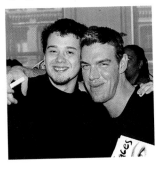

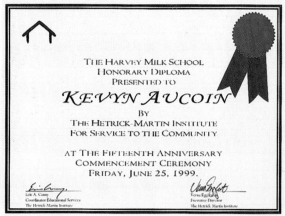

THE HARVEY MILK SCHOOL
HONORARY DIPLOMA
PRESENTED TO

KEVYN AUCOIN

BY
THE HETRICK-MARTIN INSTITUTE
FOR SERVICE TO THE COMMUNITY

AT THE FIFTEENTH ANNIVERSARY
COMMENCEMENT CEREMONY
FRIDAY, JUNE 25, 1999.

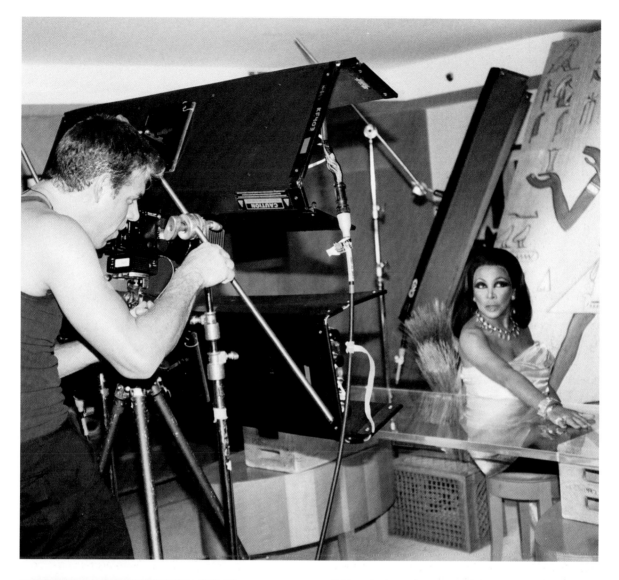

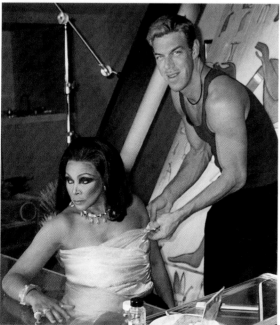

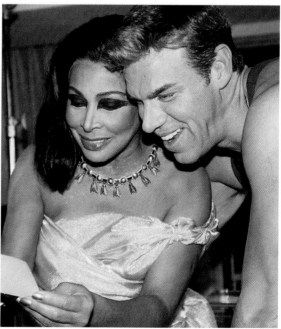

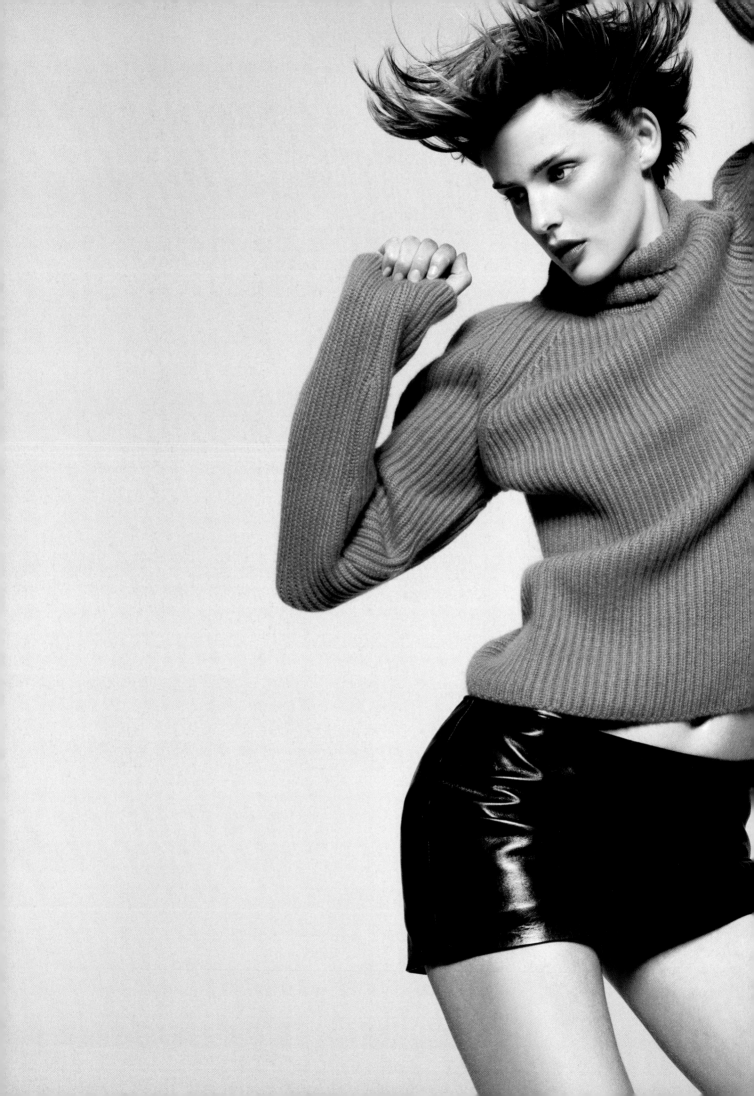

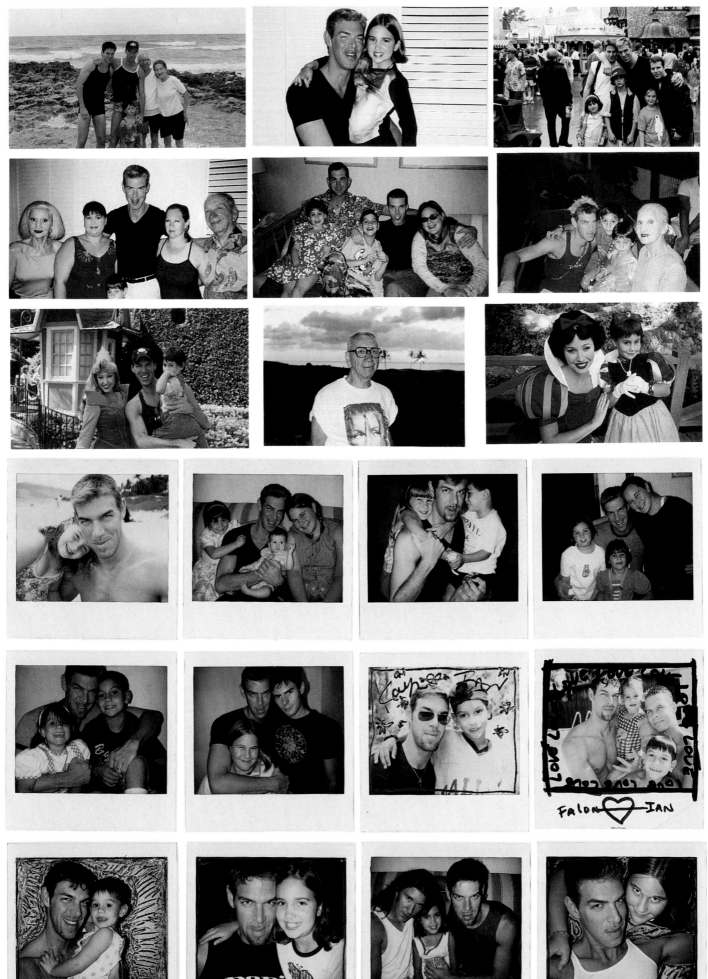

The year had been such a success, personally and professionally, that Kevyn treated his family to a weeklong vacation in Hawaii. "One thing I don't really have a lot of is time for my family, because I'm traveling so much," confessed Kevyn back then.

He was thrilled to hang out with his nieces and nephew for seven uninterrupted days. "Kevyn and the kids, oh Lord," sighs his sister Kim Trahan. "He spoiled them rotten." Kevyn turned the Aucoin family home into a toy store each Christmas, and he took each of the children to Disney World or Disneyland. "It was always 'Uncle Kevyn, Uncle Kevyn,'" continues Kim. "They loved seeing him. They'd have a blast when he was around."

Kevyn would return to Hawaii seven months later, in July 2001, to take part in a commitment ceremony with Jeremy, his boyfriend of two and a half years. Wearing leis, no shirts, and deep tans, the two exchanged rings and recited the vows they had written. "Our love is everything," said Kevyn during the ceremony. "This is a sacred promise I will not break."

Fame, as Kevyn learned, certainly had its perks, and one of his favorites was making cameo appearances in movies and on TV. Screenwriters Caroline Doyle-Karasyov and Jill Kargman included him in their fashion industry spoof, *The Intern*. "My big scene was with Gwyneth Paltrow, Andre Leon Talley [of *Vogue*], and Elizabeth Saltzman [of *Vanity Fair*]," wrote Kevyn in his *Allure* column. "I don't know if *The Intern* will come to a theater near you, but if it does, don't blink (not even once), because you might miss my big moment."

Kevyn also appeared on *Strangers with Candy* as a funeral makeup artist named Sharpei. The warped Comedy Central series was his favorite TV show, and he had practically stalked its star and creator, Amy Sedaris, until they became friends. Kevyn played himself on *Sex and the City* in the episode where Carrie takes an embarrassing tumble on the runway at a charity fashion show; he was an extra on *Will and Grace* when Cher guest-starred, and he even appeared in Ben Stiller's *Zoolander*.

His career's first controversy occurred the summer of 2000, when he took on the National Rifle Association in his *Allure* column. "Everyone knows me and sports are like the NRA and intelligence—

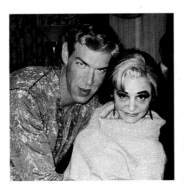

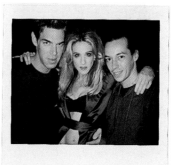

Preceding spread: Stella Tennant by Michael Thompson for *Frank* magazine.
Opposite: Kevyn with his parents, siblings, nieces, and nephew.
Left: Kevyn's script from his *Sex and the City* appearance.
Above center: Kevyn with Amy Sedaris on the set of *Strangers with Candy*.
Above right: Kevyn with Orlando Pita and Sarah Jessica Parker.

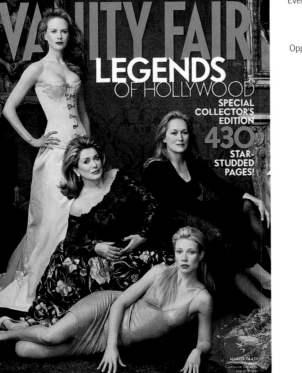

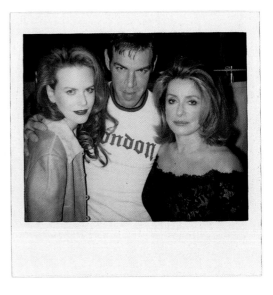

it's an oxymoron (and boy are they morons)," he wrote. *Allure* was flooded with complaints. "The resulting volume of mail suggests there are a lot of people who subscribe to both a strict interpretation of the Second Amendment and a publication that seeks to arm them with the appropriate shade of lipstick," wrote Michele Orecklin of *Time* magazine. "Among the letters were several death threats."

Kevyn was unapologetic. "The way I see it, I have a responsibility to do the most I can do, the way I know how. Since I know how to apply makeup, that's what I do, and I use it as a platform." Kevyn's acquaintances weren't surprised. "Kevyn always talked about the bigger picture, whether it was elections, abortion, or activism for AIDS," says the legendary supermodel Iman. "You never just talked to him about lipstick."

But Kevyn certainly had a lighter side that he revealed to a few of his acquaintances. "He was really funny," says Jewel, the singer-songwriter who

Kevyn befriended early in her career. "He had a tremendously sick sense of humor. I have a very dark, acerbic sense of humor, and he's one of the few people that you could get as dark with as you wanted. No joke was too disgusting for him!" Kevyn loved to share his favorite offbeat finds and was always reading lines from his *Deep Thoughts* books on photo shoots or making visitors to his Chelsea apartment watch videos of *Strangers with Candy, Mad TV,* or *French & Saunders.*

"I don't know anyone who loved to laugh more than Kevyn," says Hilary Swank. "He had such a great laugh. It just magnetized you, it was so infectious."

In 2001, almost twenty years into his career, Kevyn was still the makeup artist of choice for celebrities doing magazine covers. He did Nicole Kidman and Catherine Deneuve for Annie Leibovitz's April 2001 *Vanity Fair* cover. "Everyone wanted Kevyn to do her makeup, prompting Leibovitz to wonder what you're wondering, too:

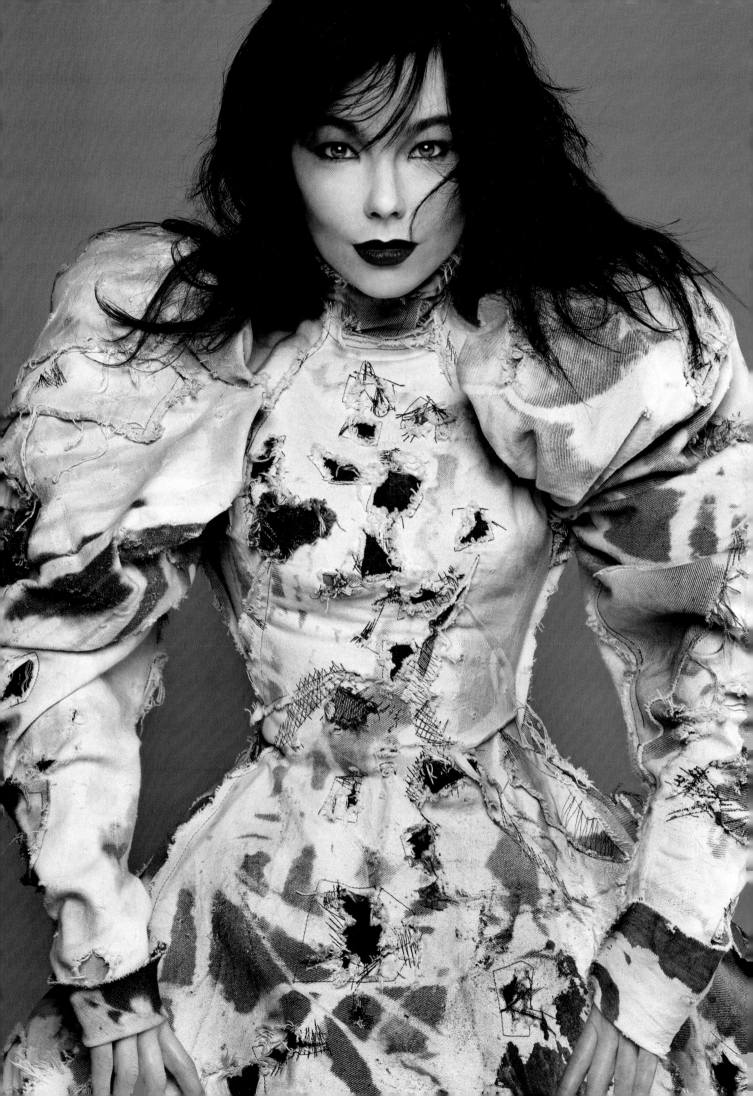

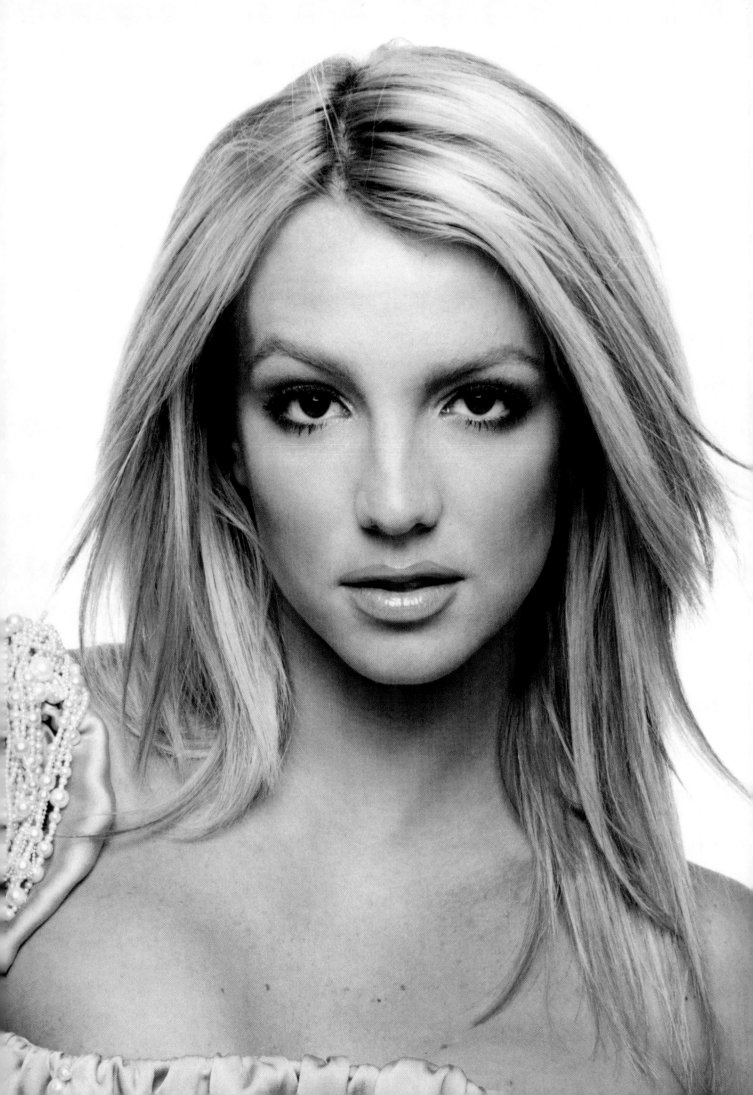

'What is it with Kevyn?'" wrote *Vanity Fair* editor in chief Graydon Carter in his monthly letter. (Meryl Streep was on the cover, too, but she didn't request Kevyn. They had never worked together, which was a huge personal disappointment. Kevyn had been a big fan since her *Sophie's Choice* days.) Then there were *Bazaar* covers with Kidman, Paltrow, Chloe Sevigny, and Britney Spears. "That was one of my favorite covers," says Spears, who also worked with Kevyn for the cover of her self-titled album. "He's one of those makeup artists who doesn't just do your face the way they envision it. He does it for *you,* too, and what looks best on you. He was so sweet and very, very nice, which is hard to find in this industry."

On September 10, 2001, Kevyn flew to Los Angeles with his makeup assistant Troy Surratt to work with Cher. Kevyn's lips had swollen, and he thought he was having an allergic reaction, so he called the hotel doctor once he checked in. The doctor happened to be a specialist in acromegaly, an extremely rare disorder in which the body produces too much growth hormone, usually because of a tumor on the pituitary gland. Kevyn had several of the symptoms—fatigue, joint pain, headaches, vision disturbance, irregular sleep patterns, abnormal growth of hands and feet, and enlarged lips, nose, and tongue—so the doctor sent him to be tested. On September 11, as the rest of the country was reeling from terrorist attacks, Kevyn was told he had tested positive. The benign tumor at the base of his brain causing the acromegaly needed to be removed.

"I remember Kevyn calling and just breaking down and crying," says Eric Sakas. "But he was hopeful and relieved that it had finally been diagnosed." Kevyn had suffered for years from the symptoms of acromegaly, especially the joint pain, vision problems, headaches, and sleep disorders. His friend Scottie Vaccaro even remembers Kevyn complaining about these things back in his teenage years. Doctors never could determine a cause, and those in Kevyn's circle attributed the problems to his grueling work schedule. Back in New York, Kevyn found a specialist who gave him two options: surgery or radiation. Kevyn opted for the surgery.

Just two weeks after his shoot, he flew to California for a *Vogue* cover with Herb Ritts and Gwyneth Paltrow. "We were in Malibu, and it was freezing cold," says Paltrow. "Kevyn wasn't so well then, but he steeled himself and did the most incredible job."

Paltrow had no idea it would be her last booking with both men. (Ritts passed away in December.)

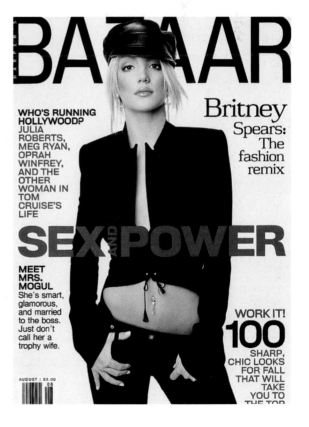

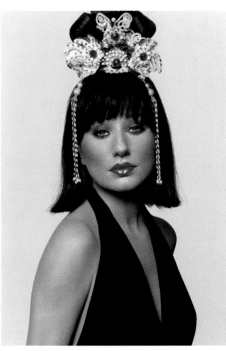
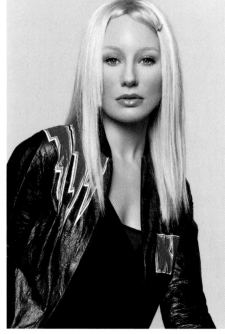
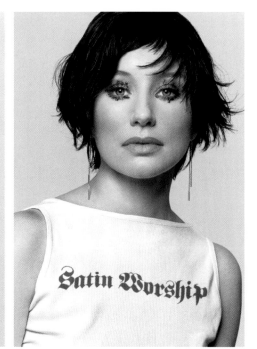
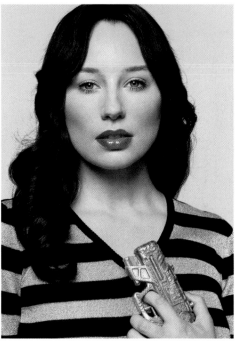
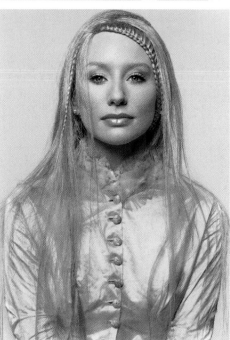
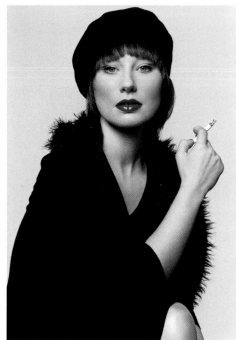
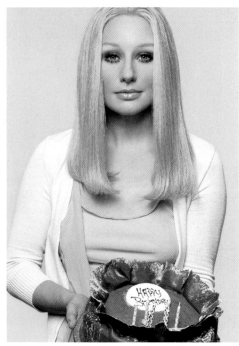
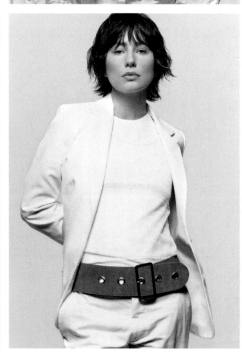
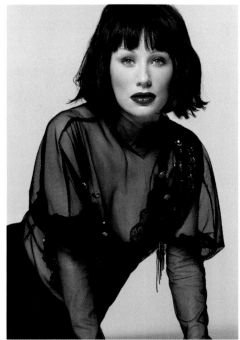

Kevyn and Tori

In September 2001, Tori Amos released *Strange Little Girls,* an album of cover songs by artists as diverse as Eminem and Lloyd Cole. Each track had been written by a man about women, and Amos wanted to add another dimension to their observations by bringing these women to life through music and photography. She teamed up with Kevyn, hairdresser Ward Stegerhoek, and stylist Karen Binns to create a persona for each song. "There was a lot of planning and back story," says Tori. "We knew where these girls lived, we knew their addresses, we knew what they ate, and we knew their sexual habits. It was that involved."

They worked on the characters for months, then shot all thirteen of them with photographer Thomas Schenk in just two days. All the pictures were featured in the booklet that came with the *Strange Little Girls* disc. Amos's favorite was the character they called Death from "Time," a Tom Waits song. "I liked the paradox about her," explains Amos.

"The thing about Death is that she's got nothing to prove. She has a lot of grace, she's seen it all, and she's very compassionate."

For Kevyn, *Strange Little Girls* was the coming together of everything he loved: music, makeup, photography, and transformations. He said it was one of the most interesting projects he had ever worked on.

In October 2002, Tori released the CD *Scarlet's Walk.* She dedicated one of the tracks, "Taxi Ride," to Kevyn. "His death brought up a lot of things in people—some lovely and some despicable and disgusting," said Tori in an interview about the song.

*I guess on days / Like this / You know who your
Friends are / Just another Dead Fag / To you that's all
Just another Light missing / On a long taxi ride / Taxi ride*

"GLAMOUR IS NOT CRUELTY.

GLAMOUR IS NOT CLOSEMINDEDNESS.

GLAMOUR IS NOT BIGOTRY OR HATRED.

GLAMOUR IS NOT SELF-CENTERDNESS.

GLAMOUR MOST OF ALL IS NOT

SELF-CONSCIOUS; IT'S NOT TRYING

REALLY HARD. IT'S JUST EXPRESSING

YOUR OWN TRUTH. I THINK THAT'S WHAT

THE ESSENCE OF GLAMOUR REALLY IS,

EXPRESSING YOUR UNIQUENESS."

—KEVYN AUCOIN

Opposite: Nicole by Patrick Demarchelier for *Harper's Bazaar*.

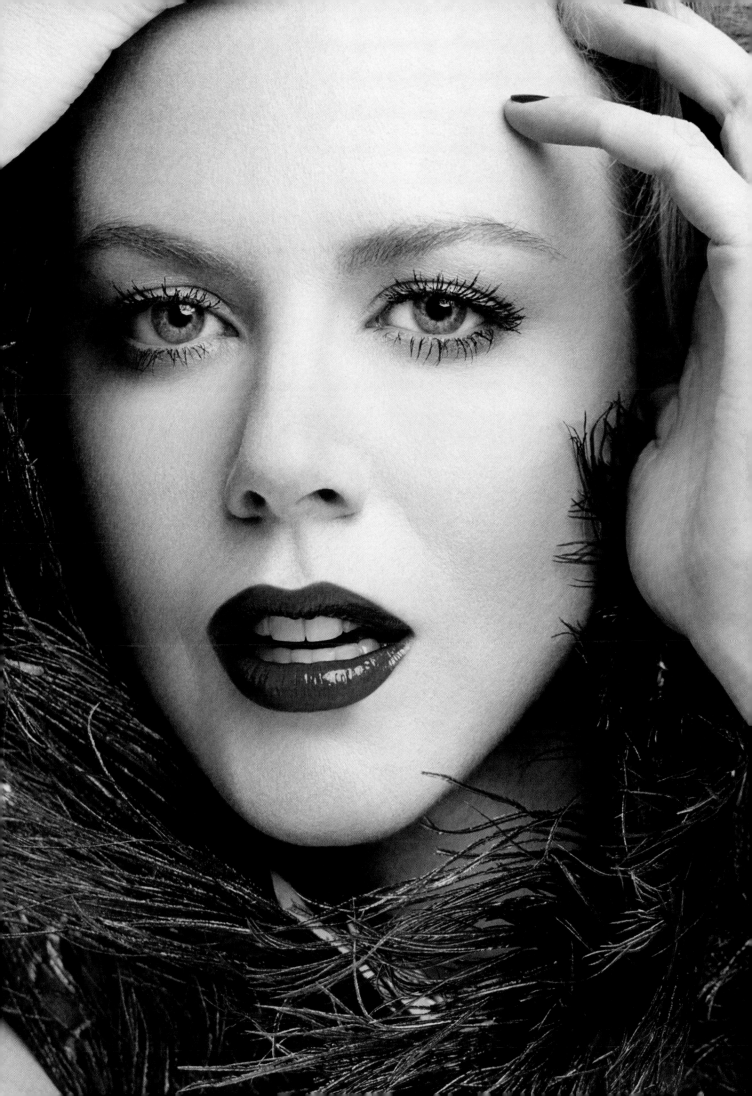

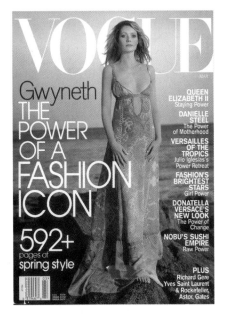

Left: Kevyn's last *Vogue* cover.

Opposite: Gwyneth by Jean-Baptiste Mondino for *Talk* magazine.

Today, she says it's difficult to look at the picture that resulted from the shoot.

As he was recovering, Kevyn also had the launch of his cosmetics collection and accompanying Web site to attend to. He had been working on the makeup line for years, testing products, formulas, and packaging until everything was perfect. He was financing it himself to make sure everything was done to his specifications. "This had been his dream for so long that he didn't want to compromise on any aspect of the line," says Eric,

who oversees the brand today as president of Kevyn Aucoin Beauty.

Rather than launch the entire line at once, an extremely expensive proposition, Kevyn introduced his brushes and his mascara first. The products were available exclusively at Henri Bendel, the lively New York specialty store, which threw a big party to celebrate the launch. Only a few people at the event knew what was going on in Kevyn's life.

But on December 9, Kevyn posted a message on his Web site regarding his condition:

Well, I've been wading through this mess alone for too long and must share it with my friends here—on Nov. 18, after approximately five weeks of being diagnosed— I had brain surgery. On Sept. 11, yes Sept. 11, I was diagnosed in L.A. with acromegaly—a human growth hormone over-production due to a tumor in my brain. It has been terrifying (I woke up—sat up—and threw up tons of blood on the operating table). I am still weak and the healing process is slow, but I'm determined to get my health back and try to find the me I've never known. You see— I've found out this tumor began around the age of nine and has steadily gotten worse. Now that I'm in the clear, I feel I can speak about this extremely rare condition. I will find out from an MRI next week if they were able to remove all of the tumor—all I ask is for your prayers and support—much love. **Kevyn**

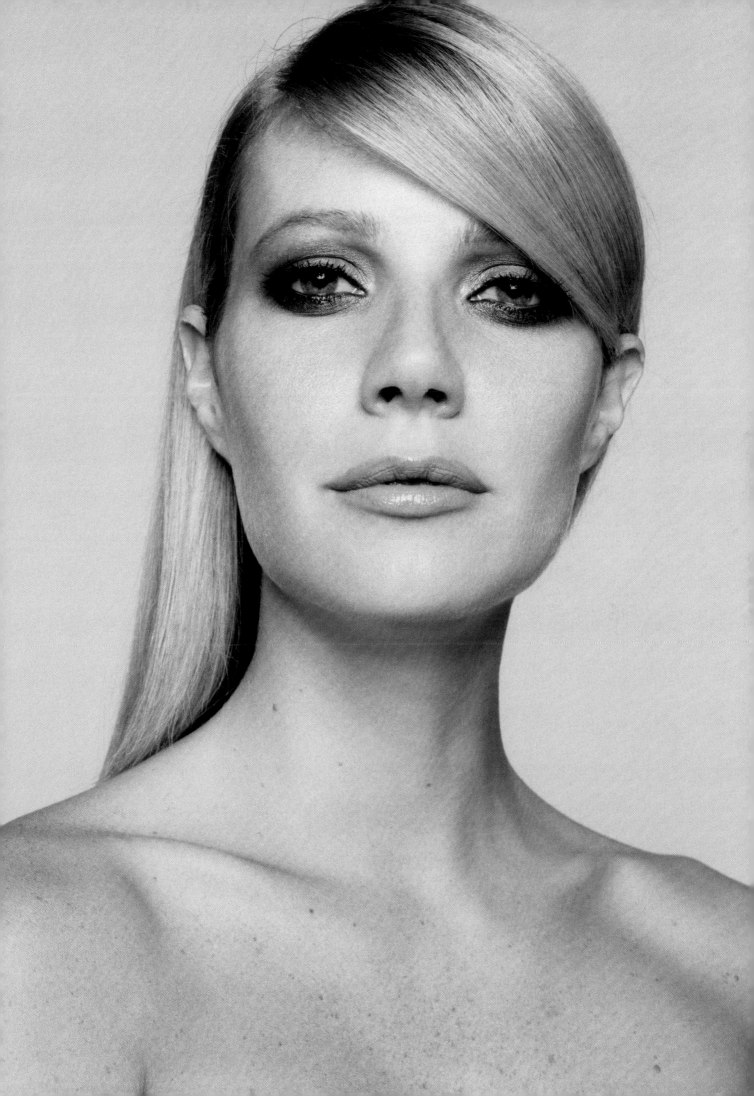

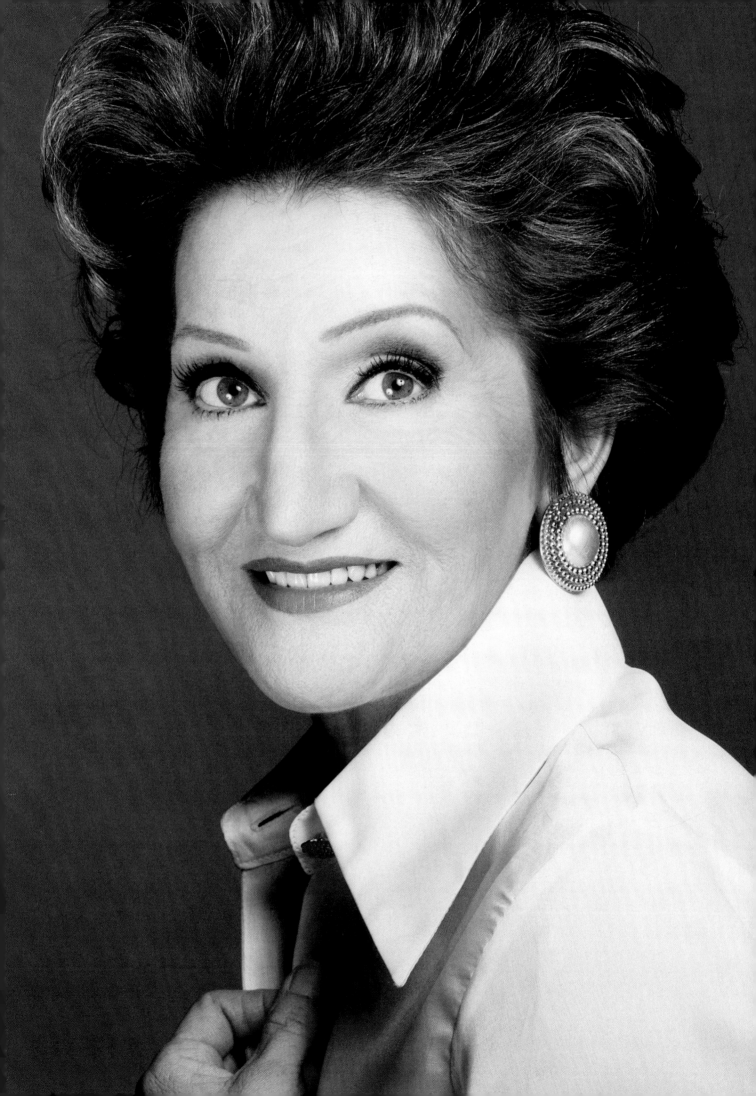

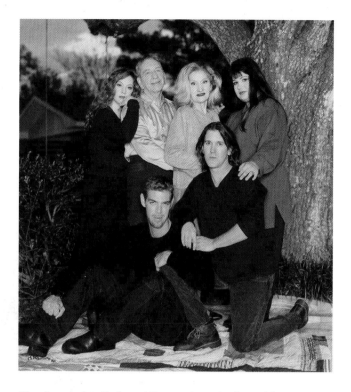

The Aucoin family found themselves dealing with another crisis just two weeks later. Again, Kevyn turned to his Web site, which was becoming more and more like his diary:

December 30

Well, my friends, one week before Christmas, my mother developed pneumonia and went into heart failure. Subsequently, she suffered a stroke and died. She was brought back and lay unconscious for three days. We spent Christmas in the hospital praying for a miracle and our prayers (much to the dismay of the doctors) have come true. Mom is home recovering with slight paralysis on her left side with a full recovery expected. When it rains it monsoons, it seems. Love to all and please pray for my mom. **Love, Kevyn**

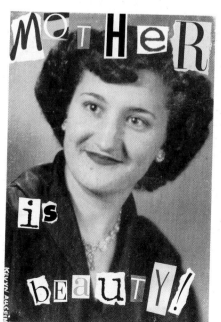

Opposite: Thelma by Michael Thompson.
Top: Aucoin family portrait. Back row: Carla, Isidore, Thelma, and Kim. Front row: Kevyn and Keith.
Right: Kevyn's collage of Thelma.

Two months after his surgery, Kevyn was in more pain than before. He became addicted to some of the medication he was taking to deal with his illness and entered a rehabilitation facility in January. He returned to the city two weeks later and continued to work.

On March 16, he did Liza Minnelli's makeup for her lavish wedding to promoter David Gest. Kevyn seemed healthier. "He looked so thin and gorgeous and sexy," says Isaac Mizrahi, who bumped into him at the star-studded event. Kevyn also did a *Bazaar* cover with Renée Zellweger and Patrick Demarchelier. "Kevyn and Renée had never worked together, and they were so excited. It was this big love fest," says Mary Alice Stephenson, *Bazaar*'s former fashion director and the stylist that day. "Kevyn seemed so vibrant and so radiant at the shoot. He still had this passion in his eyes for what he was doing." It would be Kevyn's last cover.

In April, Kevyn's doctors told him that more surgery was needed on his tumor. He wanted to explore whether alternative medicine was an option, but he never had a chance. In early May, he collapsed at his country home in upstate New York. He was taken to Westchester Medical Center, where his friends and former lovers rallied around him, but he never regained consciousness. On May 7, he was taken off his ventilator. With Jeremy and Eric at his side, Kevyn Aucoin passed away.

"The beauty industry has lost a star," wrote Ellen Tien in *The New York Times.* "Arguably, it has lost its only star." His fellow makeup artists paid tribute as well. "There's Kevyn and then there's everybody else," said Jeanine Lobell, founder of the Stila cosmetics line. "He built his fame with just his two hands."

Memorial services were held in New York and Lafayette. "God sent Kevyn here for what seems as just a moment—one brief, shining, magical moment," said his brother, Keith, during the remembrance in their hometown. "It is that special magic that will be with us always."

Later, Kevyn's friend Todd Littleton posted a message on Kevyn's Web site, hoping to provide comfort for the hundreds of shocked fans who came to the site to grieve. "Kevyn's essence, his energy is still around us, of those he loved, and those that loved him. He will be around to guide us, inspire our spirits to take risks, break molds, and make the impossible possible. I know Kevyn is still around and I can feel his love and presence stronger than ever."

About a month after his death, his friend Marcy Engelman was in her office in Manhattan, thinking about Kevyn, when she saw a ladybug fly into the room and land on the windowsill. Suddenly, she felt as if Kevyn were right beside her. She called Eric and told him what had happened. "Marcy, didn't you know?" he asked. "Kevyn called everyone he loved Ladybug."

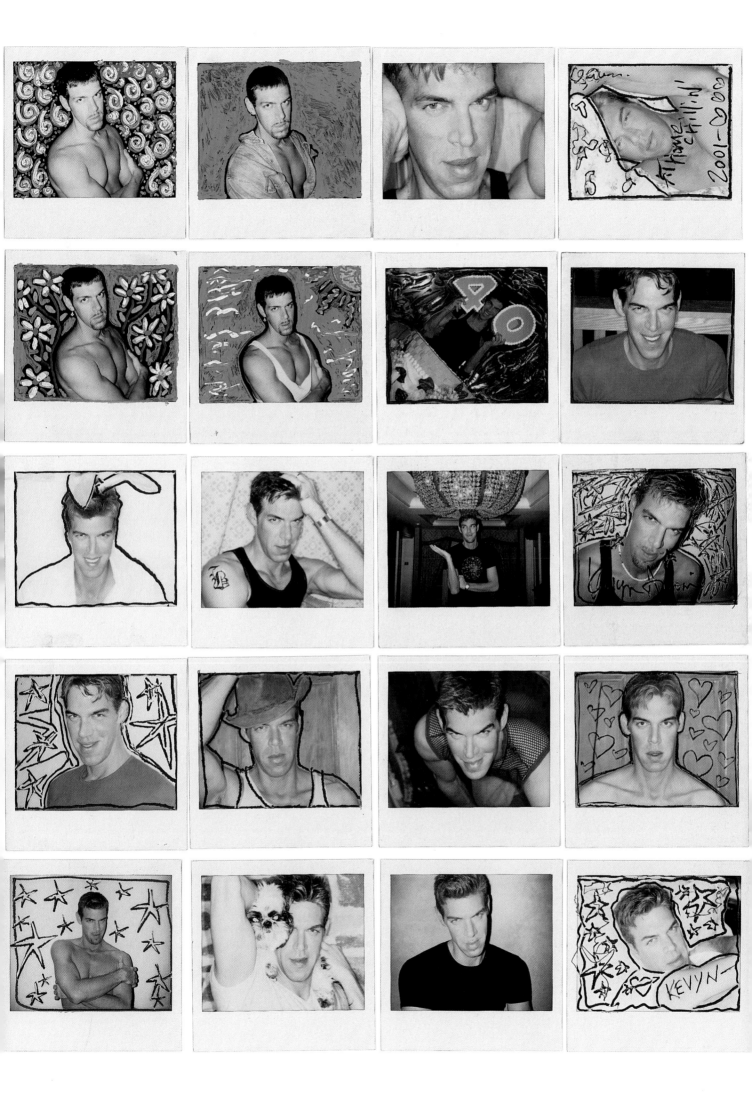

CHAPTER EIGHT

BEAUTY EVOLUTION

"When I say beautiful, I mean inside and out."

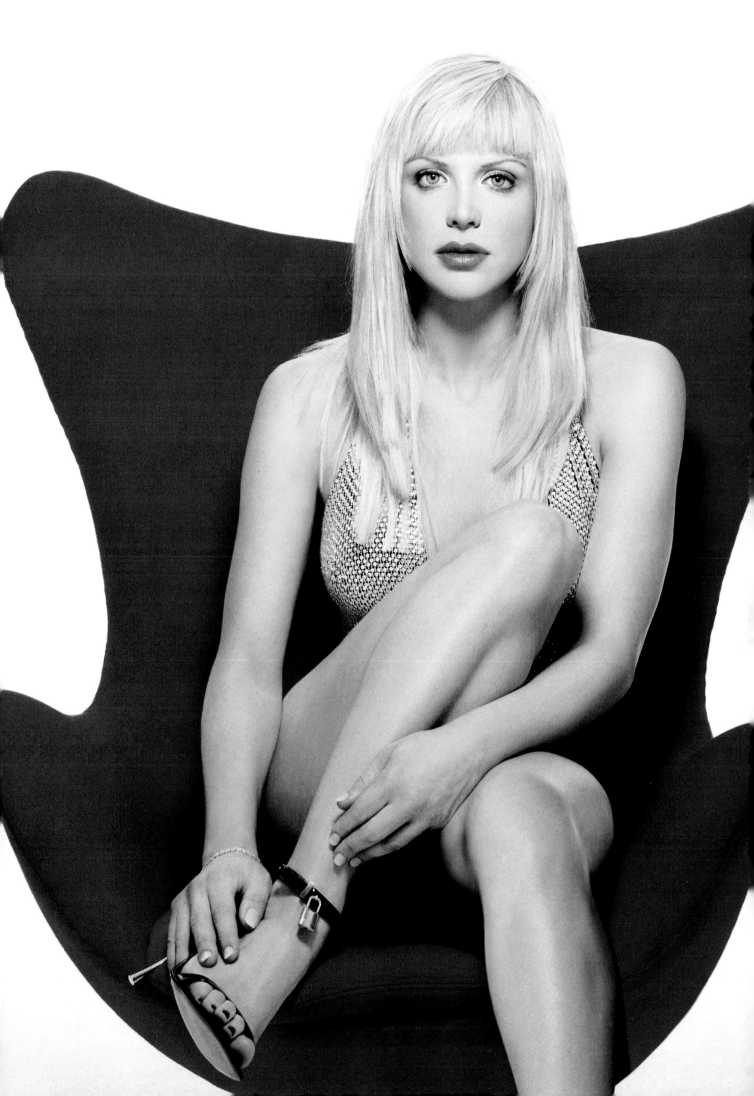

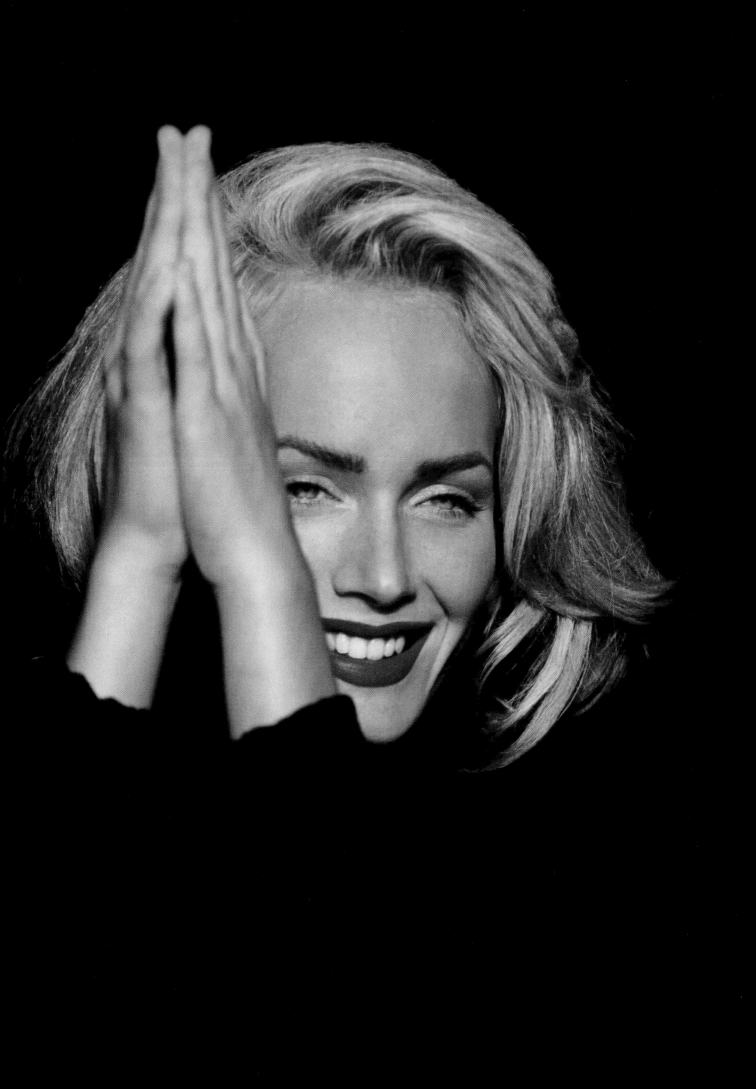

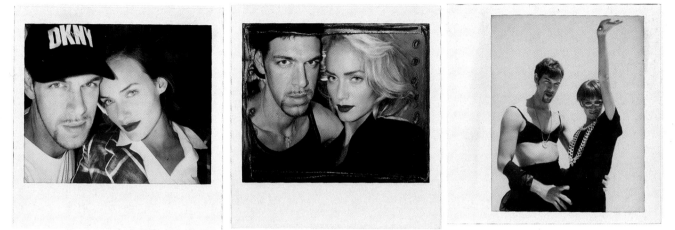

AMBER VALLETTA

Amber on Kevyn

Beauty was about empowerment for Kevyn. I can only imagine how many women he touched and how he made them feel with his message about self-respect. What Kevyn had to say always rang true because he knew different levels of pain and suffering. Often, if you're in the public eye, people don't want to hear how you feel about certain things, but you have a responsibility to have a voice and use it wisely. Kevyn did just that, and a lot of people benefited.

Kevyn on Amber

To put it simply, Amber is one of the sweetest, kindest people I have ever met in the fashion industry. I think the world of her.

When did you and Kevyn first meet?
It was an American *Vogue* beauty story with Max Vadukul. I would have been nineteen. Kevyn put one of the photos in his first book. I have short, wispy hair, the "waif" hair, in the picture, but Kevyn did this gorgeous, amazing makeup and didn't make me look like a waif at all. During the session, he told me that he had just found his birth mother and received this incredible letter from her. He also showed me his poetry and told me about his parents' involvement in a gay and lesbian support organization. It was a lot to share the first time you meet someone. It was so overwhelming but so powerful. I was really moved by him.

What was Kevyn like as a friend?
We were never just casual pals. I had been in an abusive relationship, and Kevyn was always supportive and loving. He never made me feel humiliated about my situation. He just accepted and loved me throughout it.

We never talked about work. We talked about relationships, love, and our friends and family. We got to do some amazing assignments together, but the fun part for me was goofing off with Kevyn. We

would laugh and just be really silly. We acted like kids a lot because we felt free around each other.

How did the cover of *Face Forward* come about?
We were just talking about the book, and he said, "I want you to be on the cover." Then he explained that he was going to combine one half of Kiara's face and one half of my face for the image. I was excited, but I didn't think it was going to work. Of course, when I saw the photo, it was incredible.

We loved brainstorming what character or movie star I should portray inside the book. I told him I thought it would be fun to be made up in drag. Since he had already decided to transform me into Carole Lombard, he thought the perfect opposite was Clark Gable. When Kevyn was finished, I wound up looking like a mix of Clark and my dad when he was young.

How would you like to see Kevyn remembered?
I hope people think of him as a wonderful human being who gave us so much during the short time he was here. The most important thing is not to forget him. Just because someone is gone, it doesn't mean the love dies.

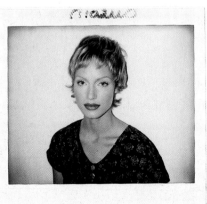 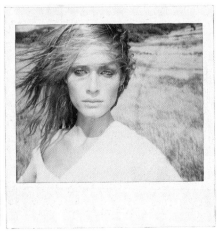

Opposite: Amber as Clark Gable and Carole Lombard, by Kevyn.

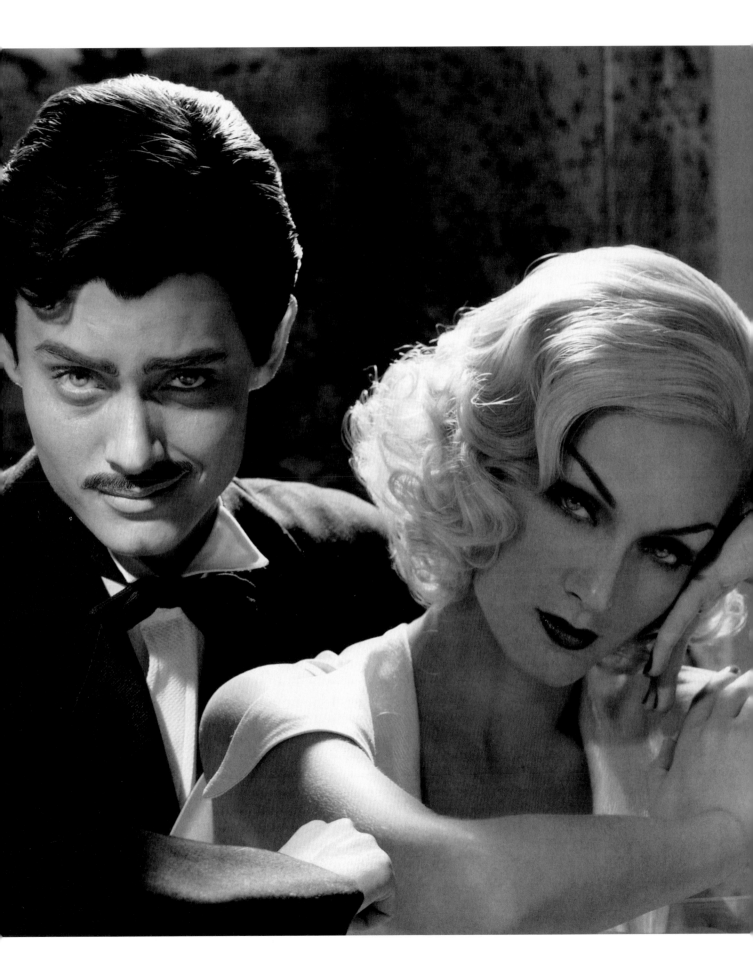

Christy on Kevyn

Kevyn was an activist and, to the best of my knowledge, this is rare among makeup artists. He was also hysterically funny. Most makeup artists try to prevent you from laughing while they work, but Kevyn was forever repeating lines from our past adventures that would make me laugh for hours.

Kevyn on Christy

Christy has a great outlook on life, and her smile does more than any makeup could.

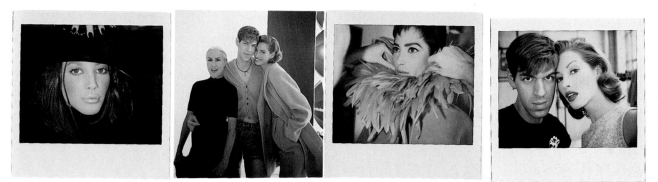

Opposite: Kevyn and Christy by Patrick Demarchelier for the cover of *The Advocate*.

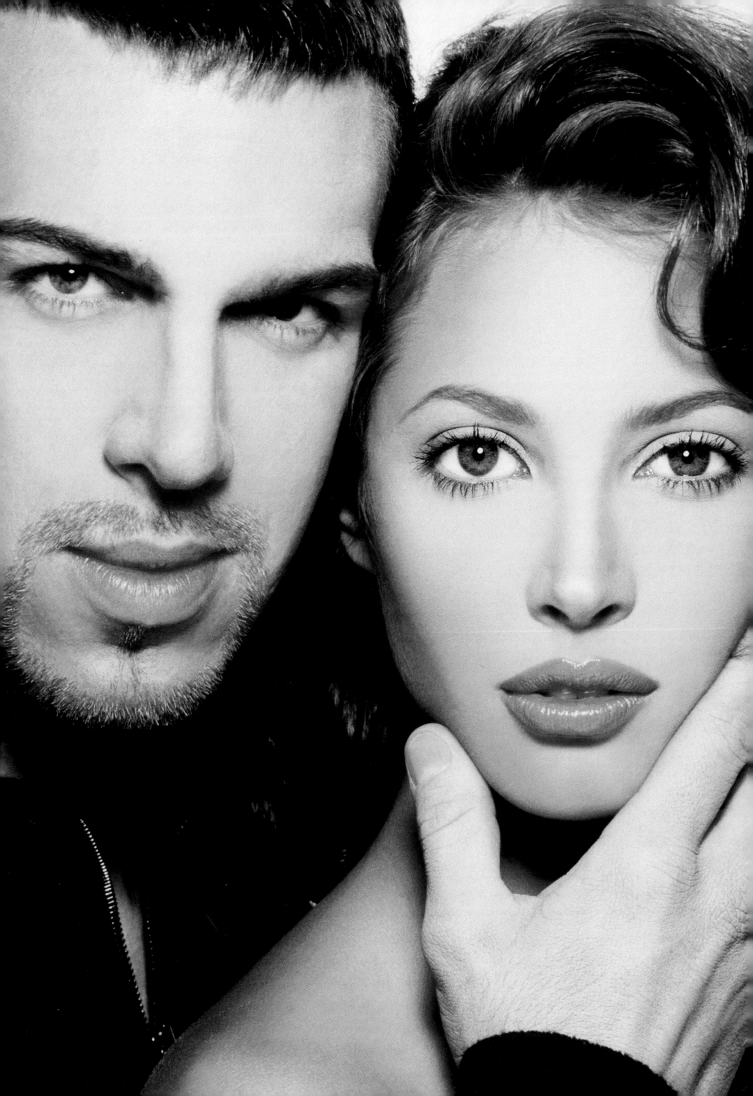

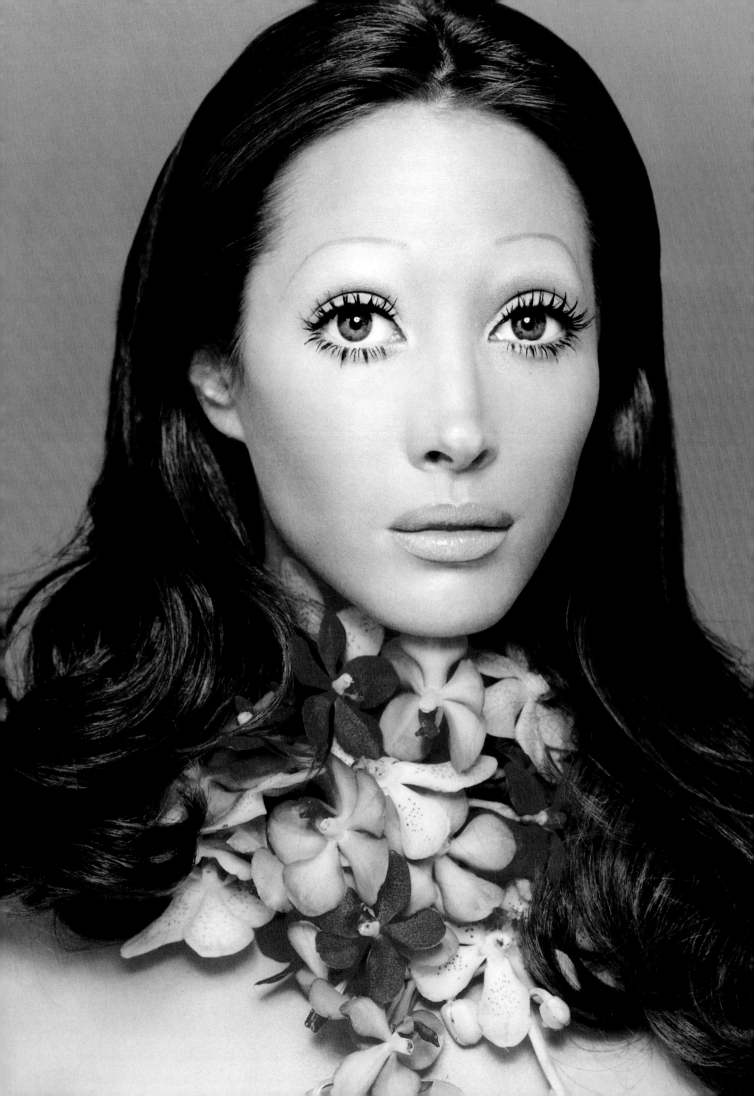

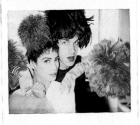

When did you first meet Kevyn?

I met Kevyn in 1985 at an American *Vogue* beauty shoot with Arthur Elgort. I was sixteen, and it was my first shoot for *Vogue.*

What was he like?

He was larger than life. Not only was he tall, but at the time he was also a platinum blond. He was twenty-three and was so confident about his work. He had a vision for the beauty story, and everything else followed suit.

What were some memorable shoots you worked on?

Every shoot with Kevyn was memorable. That first one especially, but there were many others. Once, in the late '80s, we were together in Paris to shoot the collections for *Vogue* with Mr. Penn. We would all sit around the studio waiting for the couture dresses to arrive fresh from the runways. We would then only have an hour or so to get the shot before the outfit had to be whisked off to the next magazine's shoot. During these in-between moments, and sometimes hours, we would just play. I have dozens of Polaroids from that trip that were taken of Cindy Crawford, Sam McKnight, and me. We are all wearing wigs and silly expressions in the pictures, which were probably taken at about two A.M. It was a fun time back then.

What is your favorite memory of Kevyn?

We modeled together once for a Michael Kors campaign, which was photographed by Steven Meisel. Polly Allen Mellen and Lauren Hutton were also in the campaign. Over the years Kevyn sort of blossomed physically, and it was at this shoot when I began to notice the confidence he now had in his appearance. He was wearing a tank top, cutoff shorts, and black boots in the photos. His hair was now much shorter and tousled. He was so focused during this shoot that we hardly laughed. After Kevyn died, I was moving from house to house and going through old things. I found a photo taken that day, and that is how I remember him.

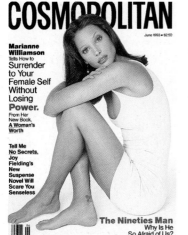
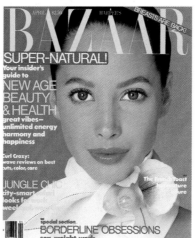
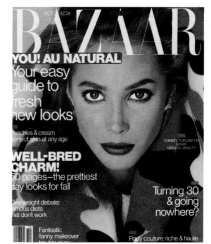

Opposite: Christy by Kevyn for *Face Forward.*

GWYNETH PALTROW

Gwyneth on Kevyn

He was so giving and open. He had such a big soul and a big heart. You felt like he saw you and appreciated you as a person. It was great to spend time with him because he was so funny, but it was his thoughtfulness and his capacity for love that helped me build a real friendship with him.

Kevyn on Gwyneth

How do you describe someone as complex, gifted, and loving as Gwyneth? Besides her obvious talent and charm, Gwyneth does what so many people in her position don't do: use their integrity to pursue a more compassionate and fulfilling life. Despite the glare of the international spotlight and being held up to indescribable standards for someone twice her age, Gwyneth handles herself with great aplomb and humor.

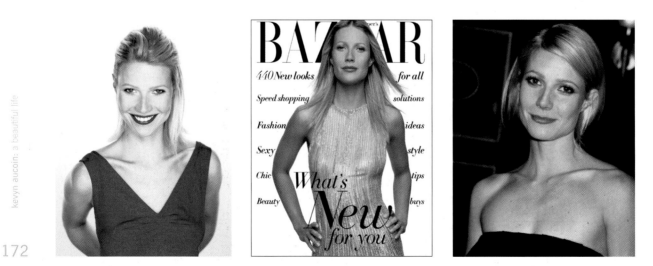

kevyn aucoin: a beautiful life

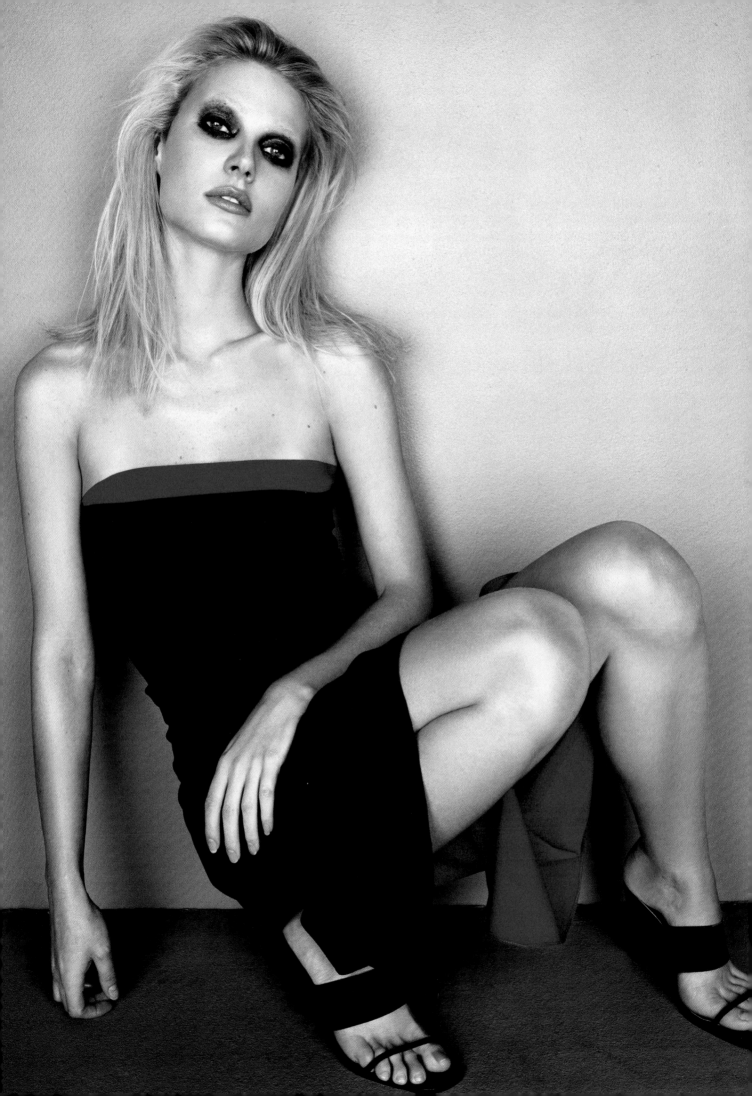

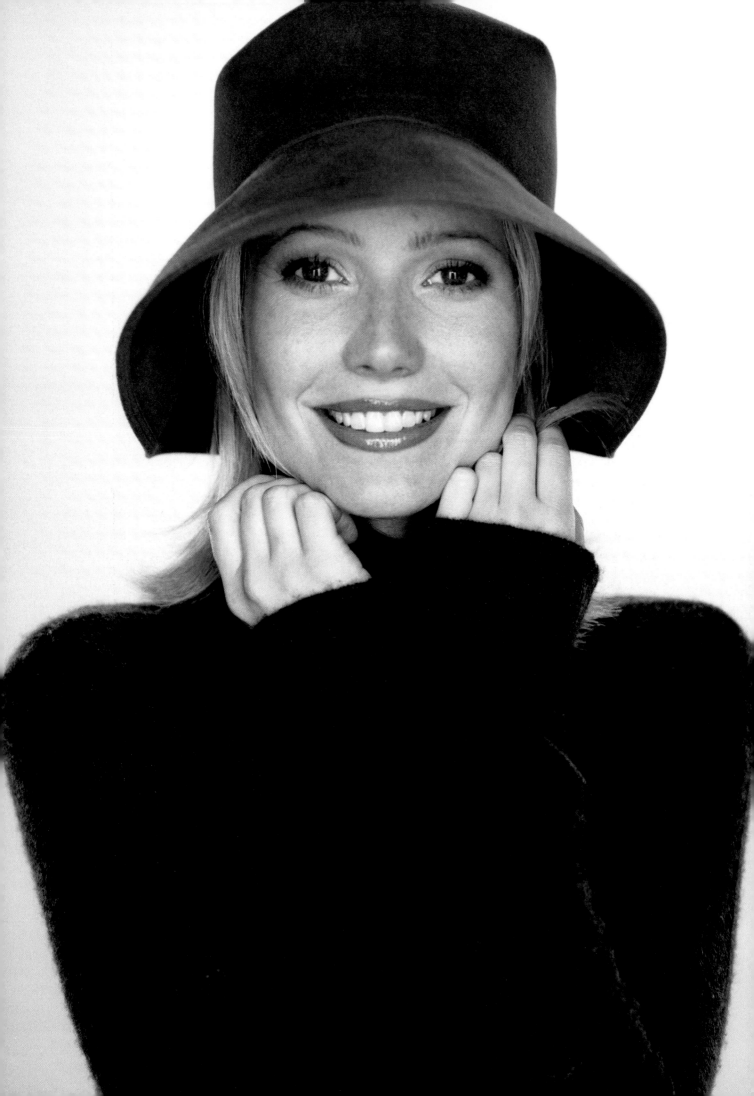

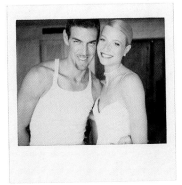

How did you and Kevyn meet?

It was on a *New York* magazine shoot, and I had just finished the movie *Emma.* I was really excited because, of course, as a teenager growing up in the city and reading *Vogue* magazine, I knew who he was. I met him, and I said, "I can't believe I get to work with you!" We laughed a lot that day. We shared an un-PC sense of humor, so we just connected. After the shoot, he gave me a signed copy of his first book, *The Art of Makeup.* Then, from that day forward, I always asked for him whenever I could. I can't remember how many times we worked together after that. Maybe hundreds.

Why was Kevyn such an asset at a photo shoot?

He always understood what the photographer was aiming for, and he could tailor a look to that mood. He was great because he would stand behind the photographer and sign to me if he saw my body at a weird angle. Like, "Move your hips slightly to the right. It's bothering me!" right behind the photographer's head.

What is your funniest memory of Kevyn?

We had just finished shooting the cover of *Harper's Bazaar* with Patrick Demarchelier in East Hampton, and it had been a really nice day. I drove Kevyn back into the city in my little Saab convertible, and we got stuck in traffic for what seemed like four hours. We were listening to Chris Rock on the CD player, and we were so delirious from just sitting in the car. It was insane. At one point, my ass fell asleep, and I was, like, "Kevyn, you have to punch me in the ass because I can't sit here anymore. I can't feel my ass." I pulled myself up on the steering wheel, turned to the side, and he started punching. We looked in the next lane, and there was this van filled with guys staring at us, like, "What the hell is going on?" We almost died. We both had to pee so badly at that point, and then we started laughing so hard. We were, like, "Oh, my God, we're going to pee in the car." It was totally classic.

Opposite: Robert Fleischauer for French *Elle.*

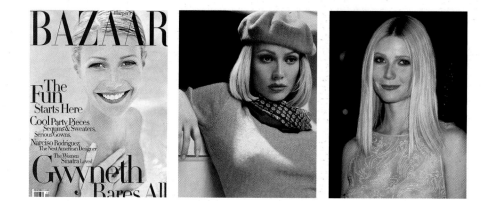

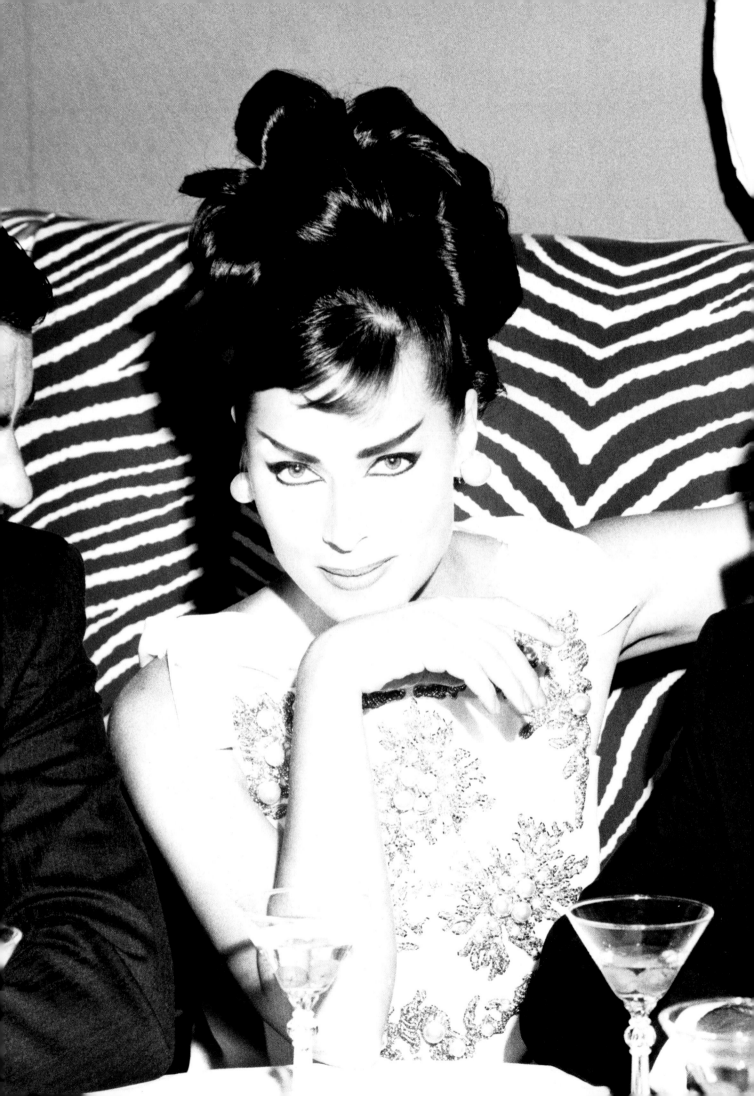

ISABELLA ROSSELLINI

Isabella on Kevyn

One day he'll discover canvas, and he'll be so happy.

Kevyn on Isabella

With this canvas, why would I want a plain old tarp?

How did Kevyn transform makeup into an art form? For Kevyn, and a few others, like Francois Nars and Laura Mercier, makeup was an instrument, the same way a brush or color is for a painter. The finished face was the expression of their talent. When I think of how Kevyn painted me, I think of Jackson Pollock and that black-and-white photo that shows him with his canvas on the floor, looking at it with a brush and the paint in his hand. His canvas was on the floor, not on an easel. When Kevyn did my makeup, he would throw me on the floor, look at me, then he

would kneel and stand, kneel and stand. Sometimes, when he stepped back to look at his work, he would squint an eye, open it, make a face, smile.

Most people don't know the names of makeup artists, but Kevyn Aucoin—everybody knew his name. It was amazing that a makeup artist could be as well known as a rock star.

What was the message behind Kevyn's work? Kevyn and I believed the same thing. You know, I could care less about makeup and which was the

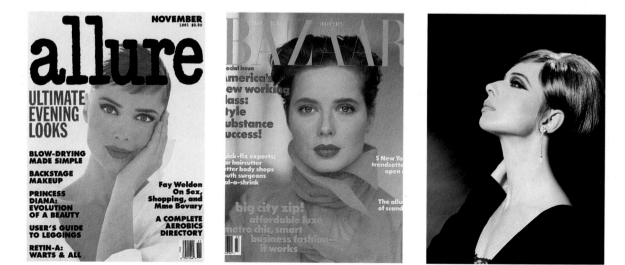

right red for the season. It wasn't at all about that. It is about being creative and playful and asserting yourself. We always talked about the exclusivity of beauty, but we were for inclusive beauty. It was a real solidarity in terms of what we wanted to promote.

Why did Kevyn love to transform his friends into other people?
He was trying to show that you can be anything you want to be. Your dreams don't have to remain a fantasy; they are reachable, possible. That probably had a lot to do with Kevyn and his personality. He came from the deep South, where he was very discriminated against for being gay. That you can overcome the odds and become what you want to be was very important for him.

Also, the transformations were homages. When Kevyn and Steven Meisel did me as Audrey Hepburn and Maria Callas, yes, it was a bit of a game. Fashion is fun, but it wasn't about Halloween. It wasn't mimicking or copying. People like Steven and Kevyn had assimilated the cultural images of the '60s and the '70s. When you talk to them, they talk about film, but they don't talk about the story. They talk about a certain frame or something very specific. That surprised me, because when I heard my parents talk about film, it was always about the story. This was a whole new way to look at films. It was a visual experience. I think there is a collective memory that belongs to all of us that is just visual. It belongs to our generation with films, television, and still photographs being part of the collective unconscious.

What was your connection regarding adoption?
I have an adopted child, and Kevyn was adopted. He was the person I would call all the time and say, "What should I say about my son?" or "What would you do regarding this or that?" I liked it because he always said the truth. He had this complete wisdom, but it wasn't conventional wisdom. As my son was growing up, I always felt that if he ran into a problem or if he felt "Why is this happening to me?" that Kevyn would be there to talk to him. So it is a big loss for me in that way.

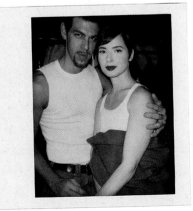

Opposite: Isabella by Kevyn for *Face Forward*.

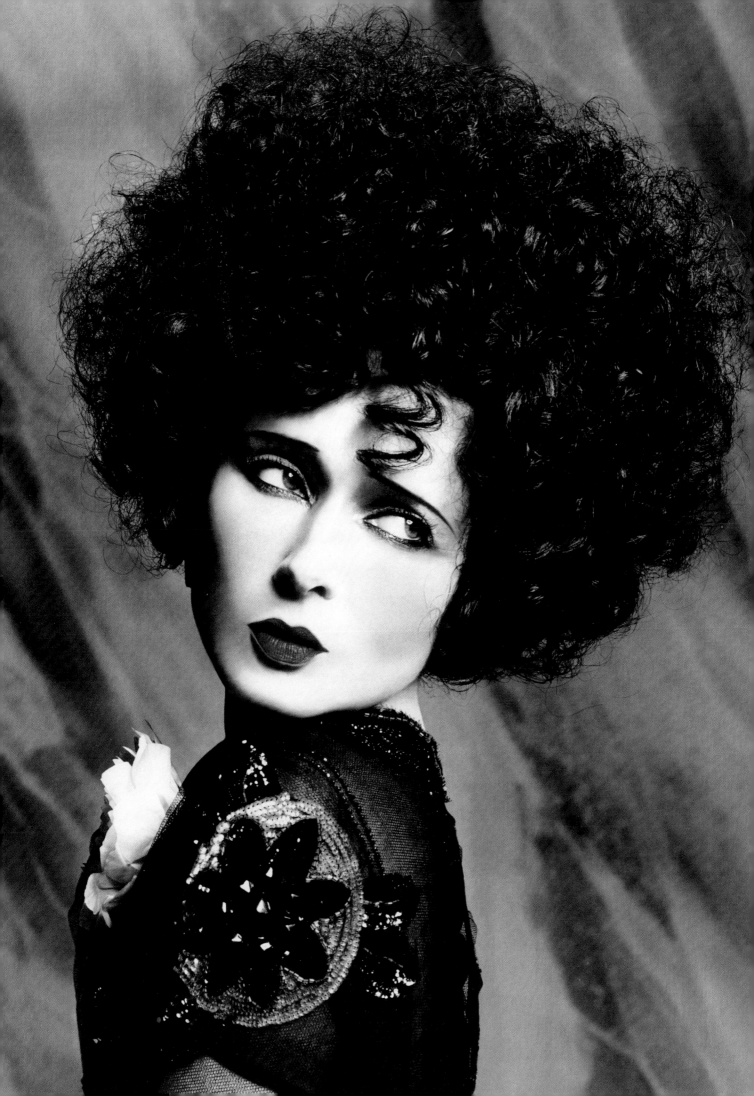

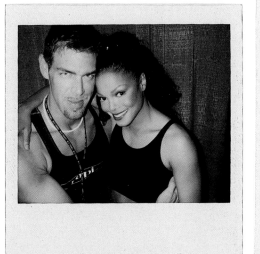

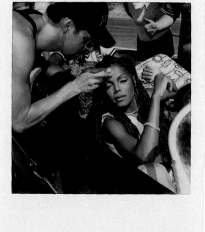

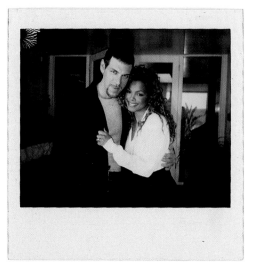

JANET JACKSON

Janet on Kevyn

I adored him. I miss him and his craziness. And I miss our talks. Sometimes we wouldn't talk for a while, and then I'd call him up or he'd call me up, and we'd just talk for hours. I grew up in a family where we were quiet, and I kept a lot of things in. He helped me to see that it's okay to open up and express yourself and that doing so will take you to new places.

Kevyn on Janet

Janet is one of the most beautiful women I've ever had the pleasure of working on. She's just so incredibly versatile. Her face takes makeup any way you want it. I can go from extremes of really smoky eyes and pale lips to really elegant, like a '50s actress, and she carries it off with great style.

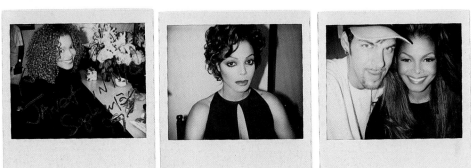

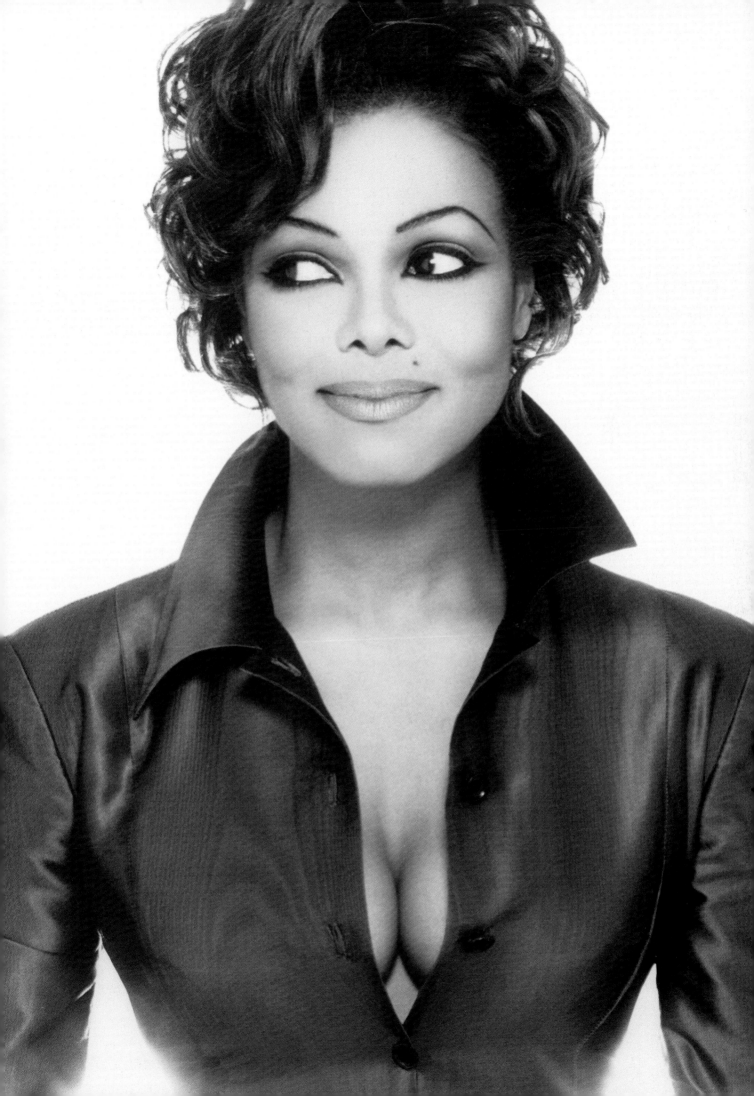

When did you and Kevyn meet?
We were in Miami getting ready to shoot the *Janet* album cover with Patrick Demarchelier. I had seen Kevyn's book and absolutely fell in love with it and wanted him for the shoot. I stepped to the edge of my trailer, and there he was, standing there, and we shook hands and talked a little bit. He became such a wonderful friend, and I fell absolutely in love with his energy and him as a person.

What was the shoot like?
I was so exhausted that Kevyn said I could lie on the floor while he did my makeup. I said, "You can do my makeup with me lying down?" and he said, "Sure, honey, go to sleep!" And I did. I just remember him nudging me, and he said, "Okay, you can wake up now." I thought he wasn't finished, so he put a mirror in front of my face. I felt so beautiful I wanted to cry.

Kevyn would do my makeup, and I know this sounds corny, but honestly, I felt like I'd been kissed by the beauty gods. I always loved the way he made my face look.

What was Kevyn like on a shoot?
He always had to pick the music! I remember one time my boyfriend and Kevyn were actually fighting over the CD player, and they were cursing at each other! We were cracking up, but they were serious. Kevyn would always bring new music to introduce me to, like Tori Amos and Eddi Reader.

When it was time to do my makeup, we would sit and talk about everything. Kevyn wrote the most amazing poems, and I would read them while he worked on me. Some of them were very spiritual, and there was definitely a deep message in all of them.

What did you and Kevyn talk about?
We'd have certain conversations about us as a people, and slavery and homosexuality. Kevyn had some very strong views. He was very smart, very bright. If he believed in something, he fought for it. I always thought that he would go on to do something else and make just as strong of a mark as he did in the makeup industry.

What did you learn from Kevyn?
He definitely helped me with my self-esteem. He would constantly tell me how he felt about me, and it would make me feel good. I hope this doesn't sound as if I think I'm beautiful, but he truly did make me feel beautiful. And I've never felt that way about myself! People might roll their eyes, but that's the way I feel about myself. He even made me notice my smile. I saw it as, "God, I have such a big mouth," and he said, "No, your smile is beautiful. You smile with your eyes." He pointed out other things that I never noticed about myself before, and I thank him for that.

Opposite: Janet by Patrick Demarchelier.

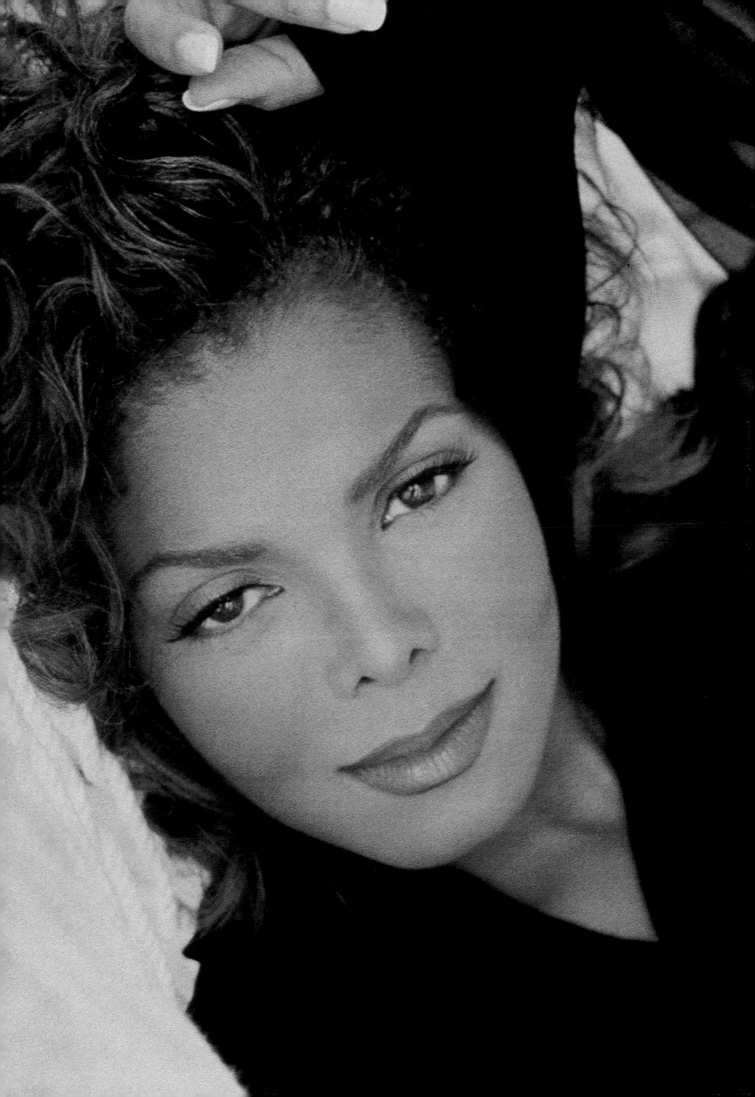

Opposite: *Julia, Studio One* by Peter Lindbergh, New York © 1995 *Harper's Bazaar* US.

JULIA ROBERTS

Julia on Kevyn

Kevyn really just embraced life. He was a great observer and was so grateful for where he was in the world. He decided to look at things that happened in his life—that others would see as adversity—as kind of enchanting happenstance. Look at how much he loved his mother. Instead of having any stigma about being adopted or lamenting that his parents didn't want him, he considered himself divinely placed with the family that chose him. He always looked at it like this remarkable thing that happened to him.

Kevyn on Julia

Julia is not only one of the funniest, most intelligent women I have ever met, but she is someone with a big heart who will show up for you in a heartbeat! She is a longtime friend who has maintained her standing in the world of celebrity with her sense of humor intact.

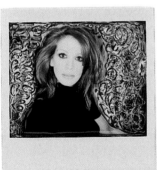 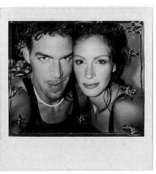 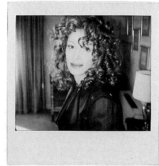 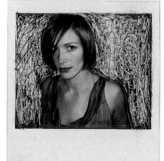

When did you first work with Kevyn?
I don't even remember life without Kevyn. Although there are pictures documenting my bad eyebrows, so certainly there was life before him. I do remember when we started working together that his big thing was to have you lie down so he could do your makeup. I think it was his way of getting a captive audience. You're lying there perfectly relaxed with him hanging in your face. Even though I hate getting my hair and makeup done, he made it great fun.

What was he like?
He just seemed bigger than life, and he was *so* funny. I guess we had a Southern bond straight off. He was so entertaining, and he had great stories.

kevyn aucoin: a beautiful life

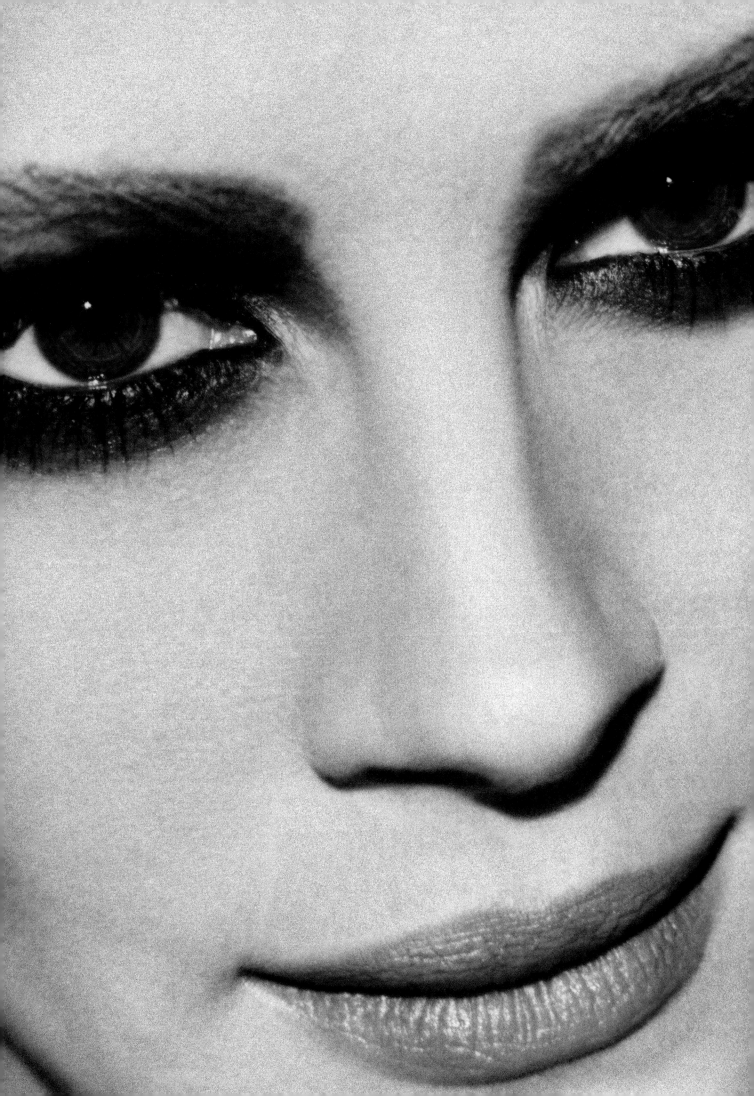

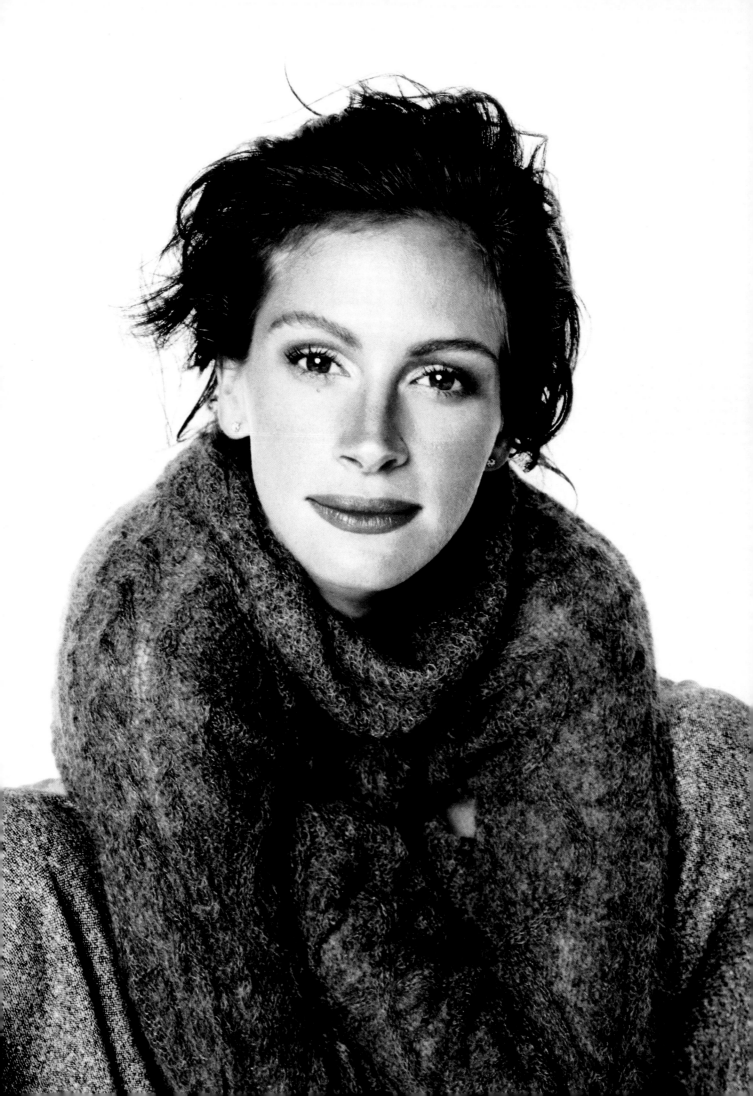

He relayed them in a way that wasn't name-dropping or inappropriate. He was just sharing the joy that he had about these people who happened to be *incredibly* famous. He was transfixing, and he was so . . . sweet.

What was the blush incident?
It was after one of my press junkets. I saw something on TV, and I called Kevyn. I was like, "I can't believe how much blush you put on me! I look like I have the biggest, reddest cheeks ever." He sent me the most hilarious apology-for-too-much-blush card. He wrote it like he was a five-year-old. He must have done it with his opposite hand, because it was like the handwriting of a serial killer.

What did Kevyn teach you about makeup?
I never wear makeup if I don't have to, but I'd say 92 percent of the products I do own came from Kevyn. Concealers and blushes and liners and eyebrow pencils and all these things. And now, of course, I can't throw any of it away. I did pick up a few tips from him. A girlfriend of mine got married on New Year's Eve at our house, and I did her makeup! At one point, I thought, "I'm trying to channel Kevyn for the biggest moment of this woman's life!" I did a lot of the things that he does, like the shimmery highlight near the inner corner of the eye. But no contouring. That's definitely out of my league. And I didn't pluck!

Was it a love/hate thing between Kevyn and your eyebrows?
That relationship, in a word, would be described as painful, because when I met Kevyn, my eyebrows were three times the size they are now. I had to endure that hand, which was like a big mitt on your face. There was no escaping it! He kind of put one hand right on your face, and with the other hand he just started pulling the hairs out. You had to have a lot of faith. But as you know, he was totally obsessed with eyebrows, so I figured mine were in capable hands. And he always did a great job.

Will there ever be another Kevyn?
Kevyn will be the next Kevyn. He'll come back as some wayward girl from Nova Scotia or something and take the world by storm.

Opposite: Julia by Sante D'Orazio for *InStyle*.
© Sante D'Orazio Studio, Inc./CORBIS OUT.

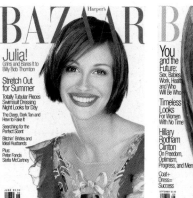
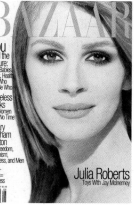

Naomi on Kevyn

Kevyn was so maternal and mothering. He always took care of everybody. If I were feeling insecure about working with a new photographer, he would guide me through it. He touched and inspired so many people, but he was always grateful and humble.

Kevyn on Naomi

What a groundbreaking beauty. Naomi helped an entire generation see that beauty comes in all colors.

NAOMI CAMPBELL

What were the fashions shows like when Kevyn was doing the makeup?

It was such an adrenaline rush because he was always excited about everything, from the eyelashes to the lip color to the shoes you were wearing. It used to get so crazy with all the paparazzi backstage and everybody throwing cameras around, hitting people in the head. Kevyn was very clear: "Excuse me, I need my light." For him, it was all about getting the girl done and getting the next one in the chair. Everyone wanted Kevyn to do their makeup, not his assistants, so you'd have to wait your turn. I waited on line for Kevyn many a time! As much as people say that I was often late, I knew

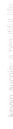

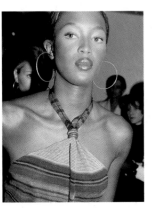 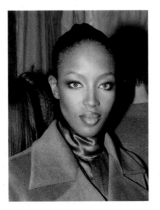 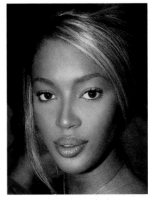

Opposite: Naomi by Michael Thompson for *Allure* © Condé Nast Publications Inc.

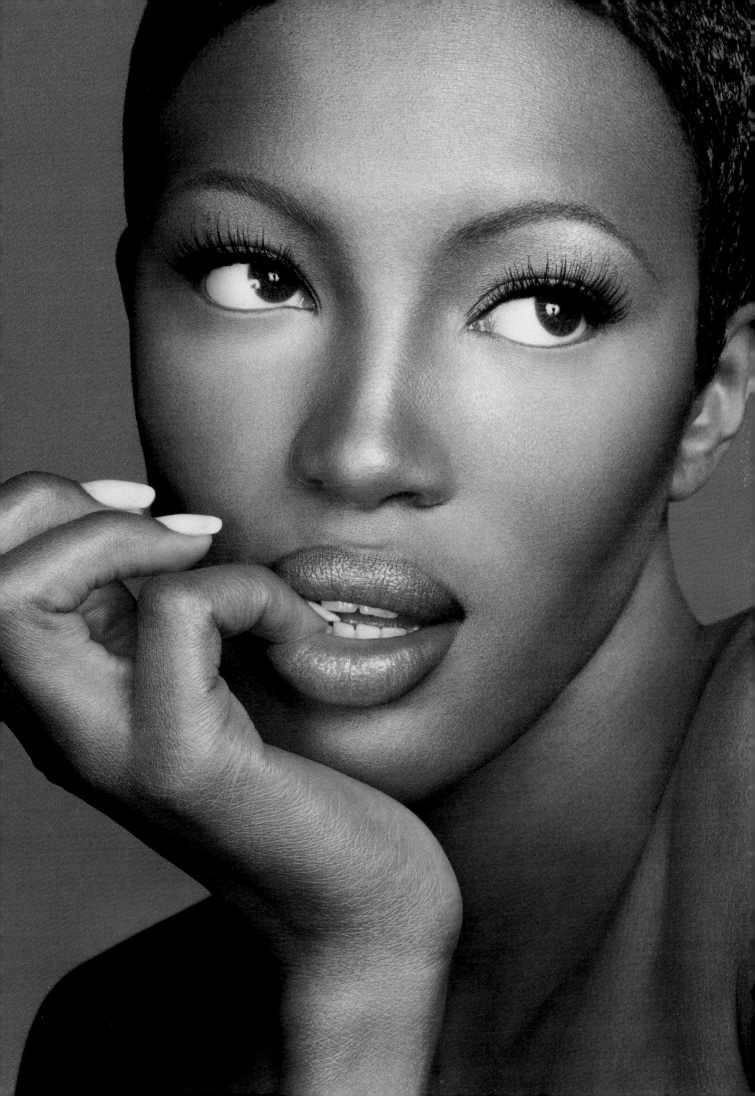

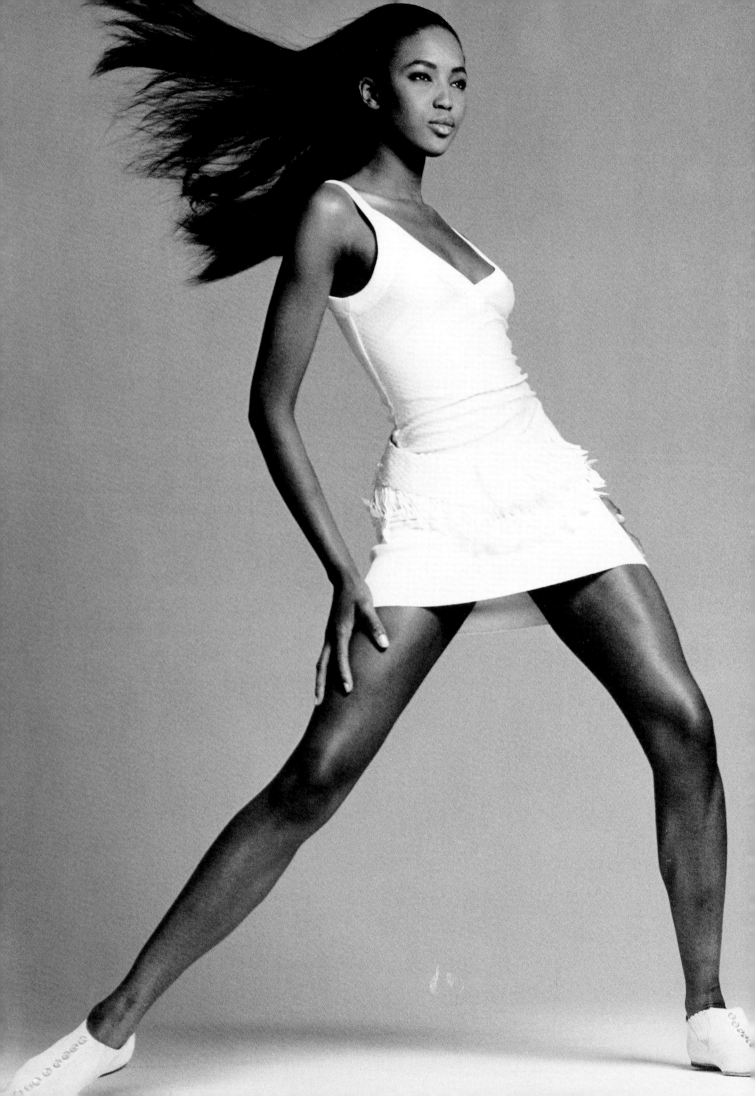

that I had to get to the show promptly if I wanted Kevyn to do my makeup.

What was it like to undergo one of Kevyn's transformations?
He could truly make you into a character. I remember when I did a job with Kevyn and Steven Meisel. We were shooting a women's ad and a men's ad for a clothing company. Steven was trying to find a male model, and then he went, "Forget it, we're going to make you the male!" They turned me into this Cuban boy, and I really looked the part. Kevyn made you believe in the fantasy and become that person. It was magic.

What are some of your favorite memories of working with Kevyn?
I loved the Isaac Mizrahi shows and Todd Oldham's. The shoot we did with Brigitte Lacombe for *Time* magazine. We had no idea it was going to be the cover. I remember working with Kevyn at Scavullo's. I really felt that was how it must have been in the '80s before I got to New York. He always had Big Macs without the burger for breakfast, and he loved to have music playing. He always had wonderful

CDs with him. There was this song he played that I loved, a Diana Ross song called "Now That You're Gone." Every time I hear that song it reminds me of Kevyn. He always knew what he wanted. He was direct, but he was always really sweet.

What was Kevyn's makeup like?
It was bulletproof. You could go to bed with it, get up, brush your teeth, powder it, and wear it again! He would put a lot of makeup on you, but he made it look like so little. And he made it look so fresh! I always wanted to know how he did it, even down to the mascara he used. It didn't matter whether he used expensive or inexpensive products; he made it look pretty, feminine, and light.

Why did Kevyn feel so strongly about diversity in magazines?
He was a pioneer, and he wanted to make things the way he thought they should be. He was very supportive of me in that respect. He really pushed for me to be in certain magazines and on certain covers. Kevyn was at the top of his profession, and he didn't want to live a lie. He told the truth, and that was brave of him.

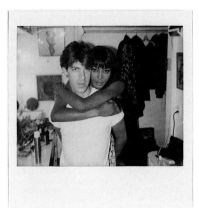

Opposite: Naomi by Francesco Scavullo.

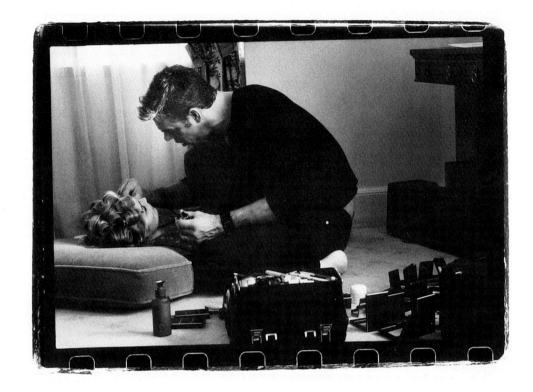

SHARON STONE

Sharon on Kevyn

I don't feel that he's gone. His presence and the power of what he's done in the world are still moving forward. He was a great human being.

Kevyn on Sharon

There are very few people who, when you see them in person, take your breath away with the sheer architectural symmetry and mathematical perfection of their face.

Above: A quiet moment. Opposite: Kevyn and Sharon by Sante D'Orazio for *InStyle*. © Sante D'Orazio Studio, Inc./CORBIS OUT.

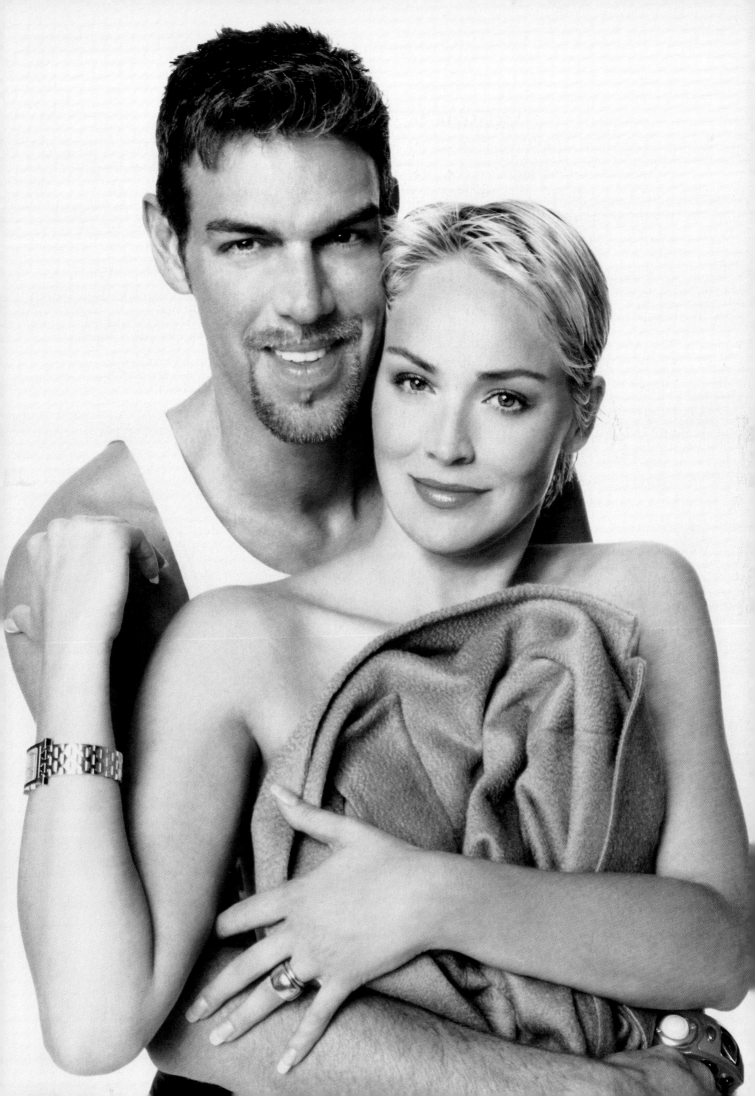

SHARON STONE

What was Kevyn's technique like?
He would come in, put some pillows and a towel on the floor, then the boom box would go down, and he'd bring out his CDs. The event was orchestrated so you could get comfortable. Because you were lying down, your facial muscles would relax, and your face would become a palette. He wasn't working against gravity; gravity was working for him, therefore he could do your face in fifteen minutes. It was just a breeze. You would talk and laugh and just have a ball. It's like a good cook. When a person cooks with love, you can taste it in the food. Kevyn was the best because he made you up with love. At the end of the day, it's all about love, and he knew that.

What made Kevyn different from other makeup artists?
Some of the supposed "big-time" people aren't kind and loving, and they think they are going to change you into something beautiful. Kevyn knew that you already were. Right from the start, he wanted to let you know that you were wonderful. That's a very special quality. Kevyn was spiritually elegant, like a great song, like a beautiful day, like a bird in flight.

What made Kevyn so outspoken on issues such as AIDS, prejudice, and homophobia?
Kevyn was just a giant person of truth. He was super-passionate, and he had wanted to mature and develop his emotions. We used to have talks about how to manage that passion so it would be influential in the most thoughtful, spiritually elegant, and profound way. For example, we'd discuss how our anger over what was and wasn't being done politically could be formed into a meaningful, useful request, not a spewing of disappointment.

What is your favorite Kevyn moment?
When he got stuck in the elevator at the Mark Hotel and we couldn't get him out. It was awful and hilarious at the same time. He was trapped for about an hour. He hated it so much. I was lying on the floor, talking through the crack in the elevator door, down the elevator shaft, trying to keep him from having a complete nervous breakdown. You know, he always tried to cram too much into each day, so he always had millions of excuses for why he was late. But this excuse was for real!

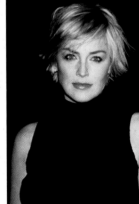
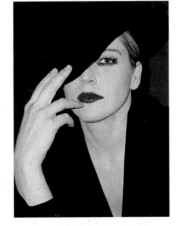
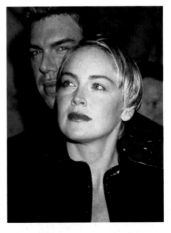

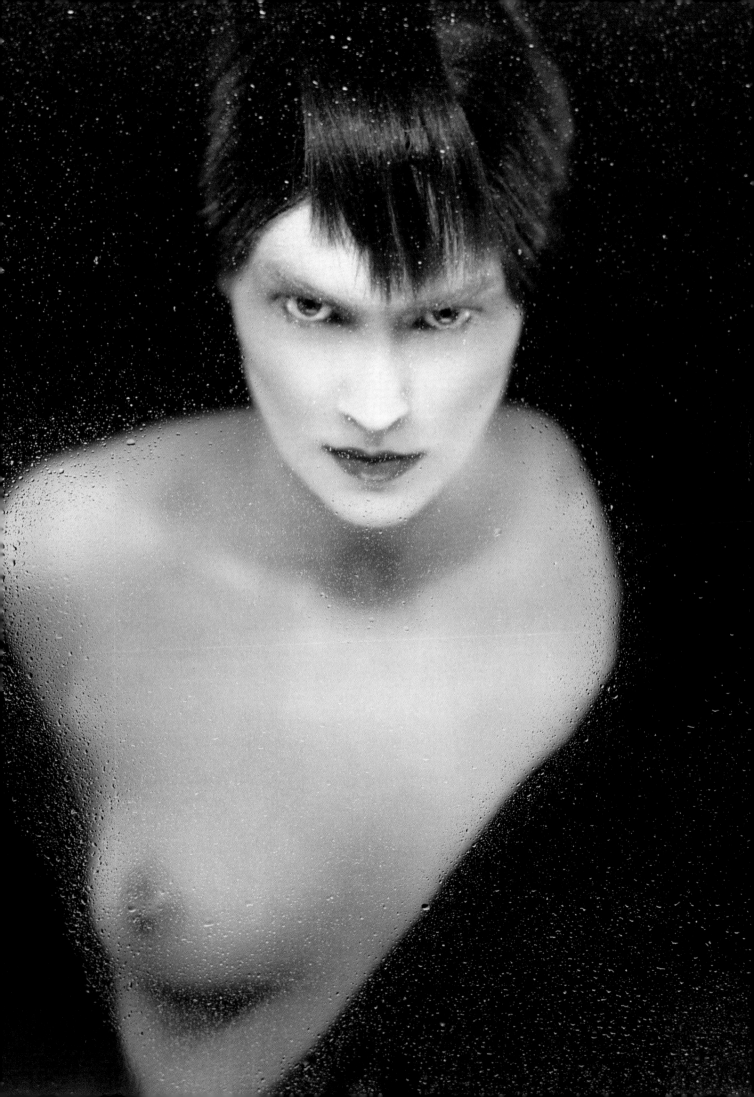

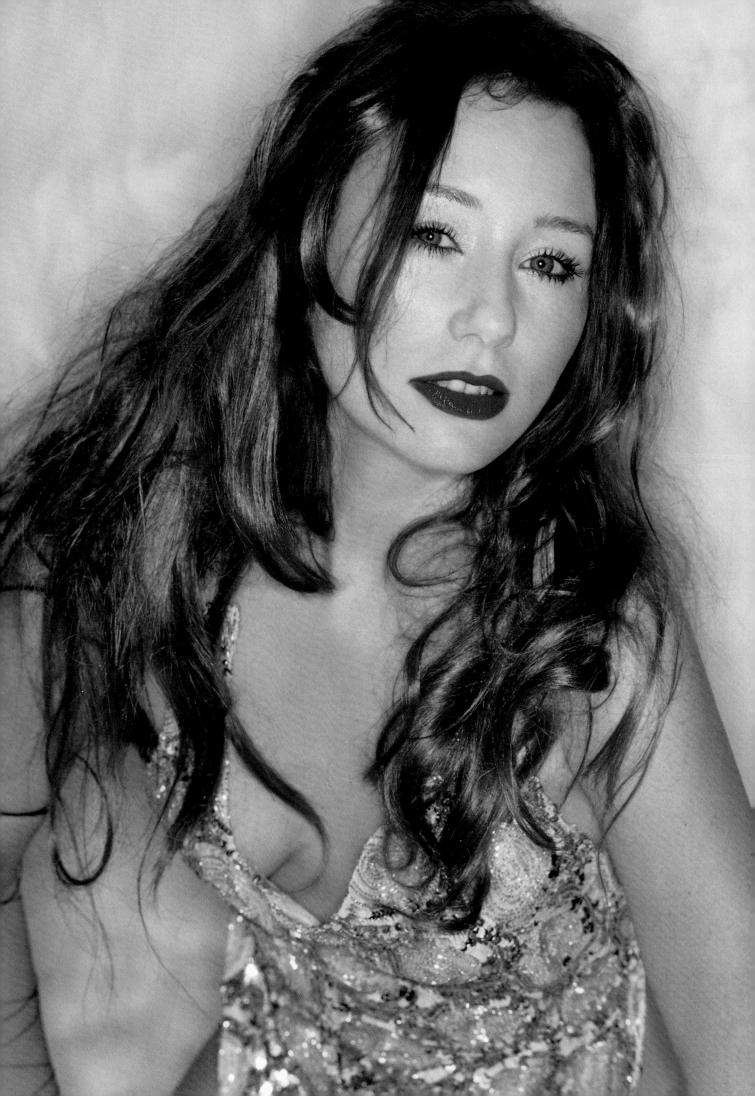

Opposite: Tori by Kevyn. This is from the photo shoot for the cover of her single, "Jackie's Strength."

Tori on Kevyn

His mind worked so fast. He was ten steps ahead of most people in the room.

Kevyn on Tori

Tori has a special understanding, not only about emotional truth but also about her makeup. I'm not talking about being pretty for a video—she understands how makeup can express a feeling, and she's the least vain person I've ever met.

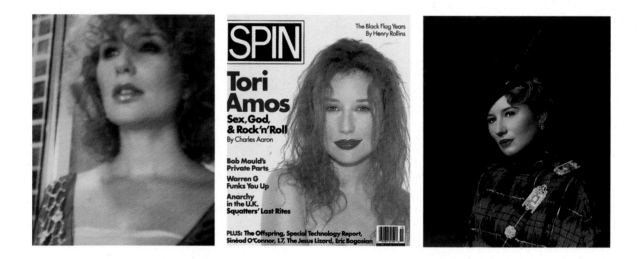

How did you and Kevyn meet?
I think it was years ago on a shoot for *Rolling Stone.* He always searched people out, which is so funny because he didn't have to. I was a new artist at the time, and I didn't even know that a makeup artist of his stature—and his price tag—would be available to me. Kevyn cut a deal on his rate so he could do the shoot. And then our friendship began.

What was it like to have Kevyn do your makeup?
He always tried to bring something out in you when he did your makeup. You would walk in, you're not feeling well, and he shows you something in yourself. Then somehow his makeup would reflect and accentuate that quality. He could do that with anybody, even with people you wouldn't want to spend more than five minutes with your whole life. Then

Opposite: Tori by Thomas Schenk as "Happiness Is a Warm Gun" from her *Strange Little Girls* CD.

you would go onstage or on television or whatever, and the thing that he saw in you is what you'd take and project in front of all these people.

Tell me about his relationship with music.
He would always be playing music. All the time. When I would see him, he would always turn me on to something new. Turning artists on to other artists was a real passion of his. There are a lot of artists who never meet each other because you're touring all the time and things can get very competitive in the music business, just because of how the industry pits you against each other. He was always trying to break that down.

Why did you work well together?
I would never look at music the way he did. He could always bring something to a project just because of his visual sense about music. I don't mean about what you're wearing or what you're

looking like. I'm talking about how the music made him see and what it made him see.

He was a part of my think tank. I've always had a handful of people in every different field that I would play my music for before anybody else heard it. And they would say, "Well, hey, did you think about this?" or "This is what I kind of didn't get from it, and this is what I did get from it." I would go back to the woodshed for a few months, then play it for them again.

What did you love about Kevyn?
He never judged people about what they were going through. He could be wickedly funny and say things like, "So, who's on diet pills this week?" But he's not one of those people who would ditch you. There are very few people who deserved his friendship. I don't even know if I did, really. His friendship was that deep.

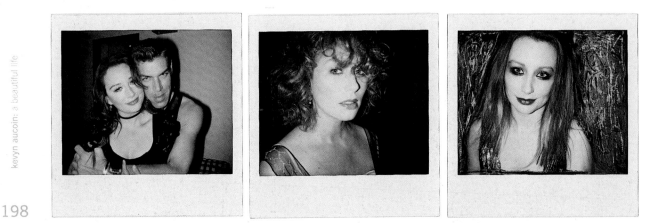

"Today I see beauty everywhere I go, in every face I see, in every single soul, and sometimes even in myself."

CHAPTER NINE

ESSENTIAL AUCOIN:
KEVYN'S BEST BEAUTY ADVICE

Opposite: Ashley Judd by Patrick Demarchelier for *Harper's Bazaar*.

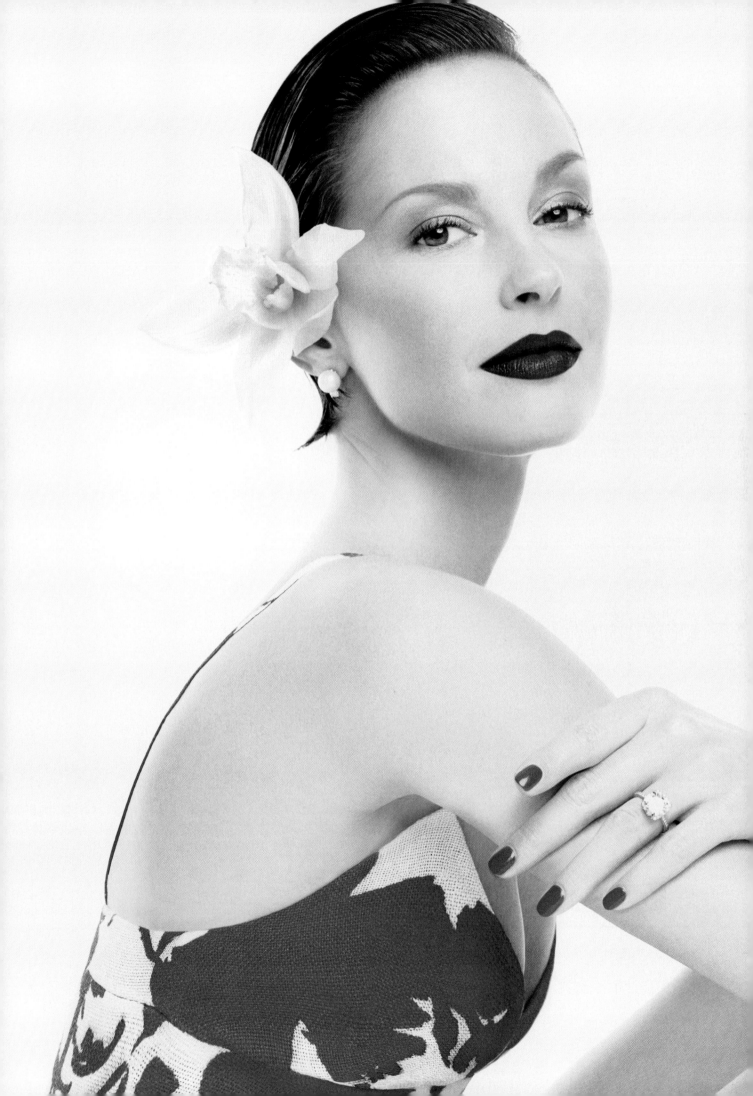

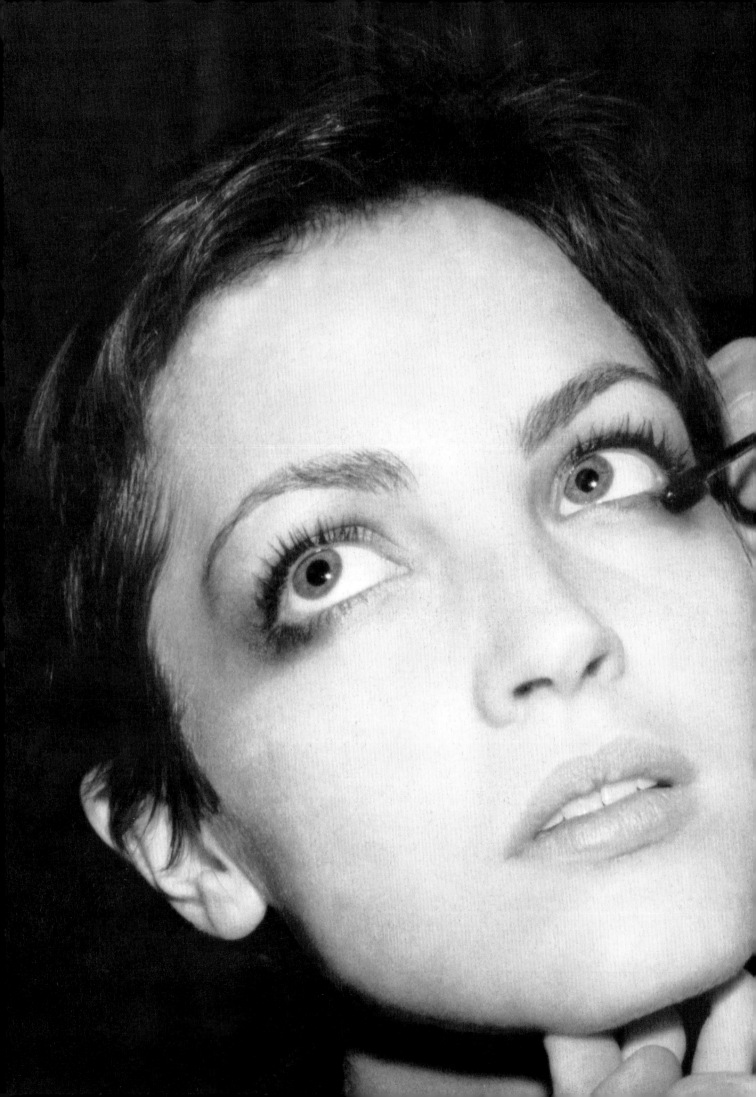

"EVERYONE HAS THE POTENTIAL TO LOOK BEAUTIFUL."

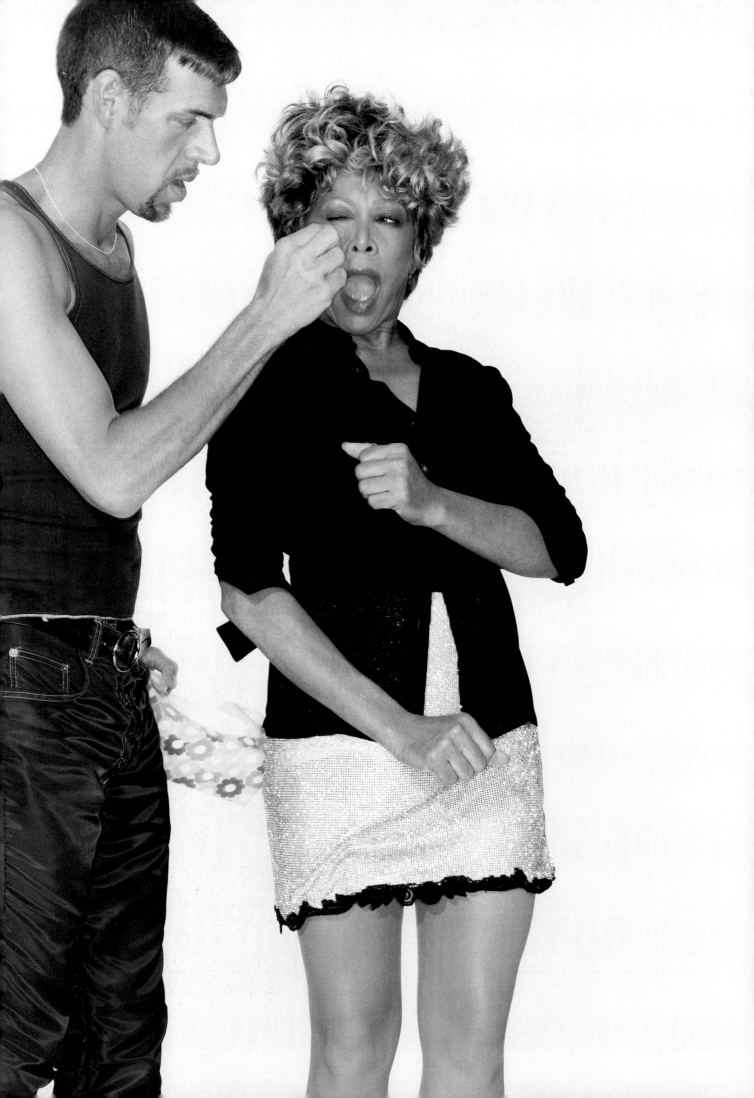

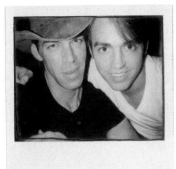

Kevyn was a true master of his craft. He could create a soft, pretty look using only a single color, or he could transform a face with a palette of dramatic hues. He would arrive at a shoot lugging his Shu Uemura case filled to the brim with the hundreds of brushes, tools, tubes, pots, and powders he used to turn even the most celebrated beauties into something extraordinary. It wasn't the products that provided the magic—it was Kevyn's technique, which he had been developing and refining since he was eleven years old, making up his little sister Carla in the family's living room.

Kevyn would adapt his favorite methods depending on the model, musician, or movie star he was working with that day. "Every face was unique to Kevyn," says Troy Surratt, the makeup artist who often assisted Kevyn on shoots. "He approached everyone as an individual."

Turn the page to learn Kevyn's "greatest hits," the tips and tricks he used most often from his repertoire. Have fun with his advice, and see what works best for you. "Play up what you have," he said. "Express your uniqueness."

Kevyn suggested that the best way to understand your own face is to do someone else's makeup. So grab a willing accomplice, and break out the beauty products, but first, banish the word *mistake* from your vocabulary. As Kevyn always said, if you don't love the look, simply wash it off and start again. Ultimately, it's what's behind the makeup that really matters. "True beauty is always there," said Kevyn, "from the day we're born."

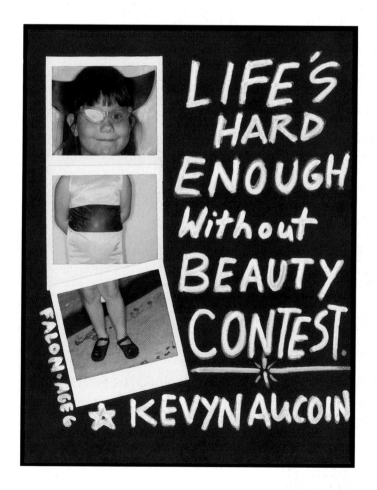

Preceding spread: Kevyn and Chandra by Eric Sakas.
Opposite: Kevyn touches up Tina Turner on set; photo by Gilles Bensimon for American *Elle*.
Top: Kevyn and makeup artist Troy Surratt.
Right: Kevyn's collage of his niece, Falon.

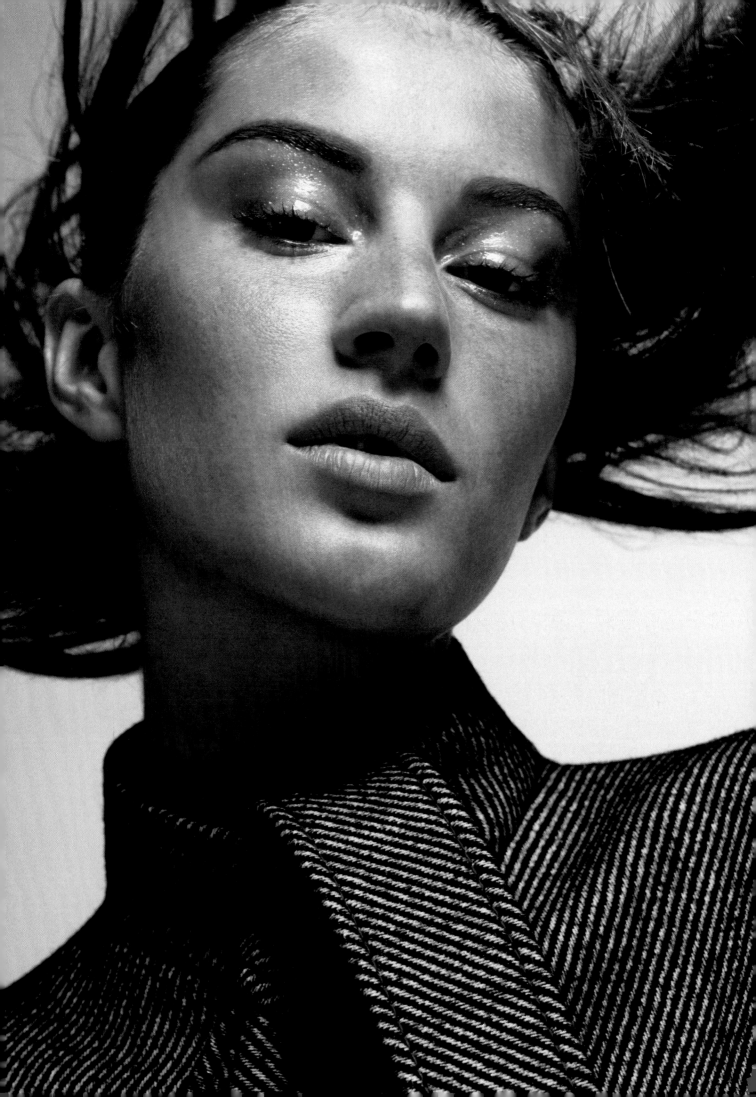

FACE

> "Kevyn taught me how to contour my nose. I've tried it when I do my own makeup, but I can never make it look like Kevyn did!" **Britney Spears**

Getting Started Kevyn prepped the face with moisturizer to help "plump up" the skin before applying any makeup. (He loved Crème de la Mer and Kiehl's Imperiale Repairateur Moisturizing Masque.) He let the moisturizer sink in, then blotted the face with tissues to remove any shine. (Use the cheap kind. Expensive tissues loaded with aloe and other extras will leave fuzz all over the face.)

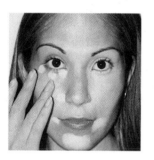

Step 1: Concealer Kevyn applied creamy, opaque concealer with his fingers under and around the eyes, on the sides of the nostrils, on the sides of the mouth, and on the chin. (He found that thin, liquidy formulas don't provide enough coverage for dark circles, redness, and blemishes.) Then he lightly blended the product with his ring finger. You can use a sponge if you prefer. For blemishes or any spots that needed covering up, Kevyn used a small concealer brush to apply the product, then blended lightly with the brush or by tapping with his finger.

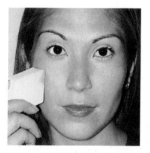

Step 2: Foundation Not everyone needs foundation. Kevyn skipped this step when concealer was enough to even out the skin tone. But when he did use it, he dabbed the product onto the forehead, cheeks, jawline, chin, and neck using his fingers or his favorite diamond-shaped sponges, then gently blended it into the skin.

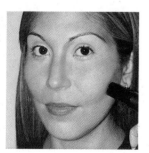

Step 3: Contouring Kevyn loved this trick as a way to define and sculpt the face. (Contouring adds shadows, which makes parts of the face recede; highlighting, or adding light, brings them forward.) After he applied foundation, he would take a taupe-colored contour stick (or something darker, depending on skin tone) and draw lines along the sides of the nose, under the tip of the nose, on the temples, under the cheekbones, and under the chin. Blending is key here, so Kevyn diffused the lines with a sponge or his fingers.

kevyn aucoin: a beautiful life

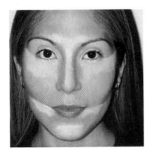

Step 4: Highlighting

To emphasize parts of the face, Kevyn used a product a shade lighter than the subject's skin tone. (You can try this with concealer, powder, cream-to-powder foundation, or stick foundation.) He dotted the product on the high points of the cheekbones, on the center of the forehead, along the bridge of the nose, on the tip of the chin, and under the cheekline, then blended with his fingers or a sponge.

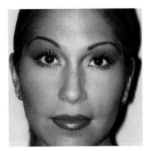

Step 5: Final Touch

If Kevyn wanted a matte or a finished look, he used a circular sponge and patted a bit of loose translucent powder under the eyes, between the brows, down the nose, and on the chin. Then he curved the sponge around his finger and pressed the powder into the skin with a rolling motion. (Imagine that you're giving a fingerprint where you roll and lift the finger.) This helped makeup last all day.

For a dewy look, Kevyn skipped powder and just blotted the foundation gently with a tissue to remove extra shine.

How to Avoid Cakey-Looking Makeup

• **Use creamy products (concealer, foundation, contouring stick, highlighting cream, cream blush, gel blush, or liquid blush) first, followed by powder and/or powder blush. Powder sets cream products and enhances your makeup's staying power. Cream on top of powder creates a cakey-looking finish.**
• **Make sure to moisturize and exfoliate (gently, with a scrub or washcloth) if you're prone to flaky skin.**
• **The problem might be your moisturizer. Some formulas, especially those packed with special anti-aging ingredients, don't allow concealer or foundation to blend nicely into the skin. You might want to save those for nighttime and use a basic day moisturizer instead.**

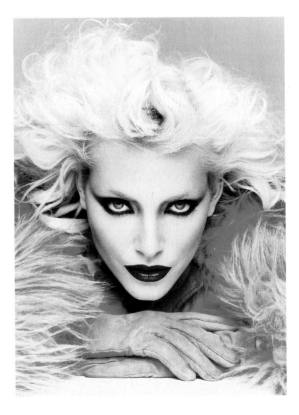

Kevyn's Favorite Tools
• Moisturizer • Concealer • Foundation • Contouring stick • Powder • Concealer brush • Diamond-shaped sponges • Circular sponges • Tissues

Opposite: Chandra by Kevyn.

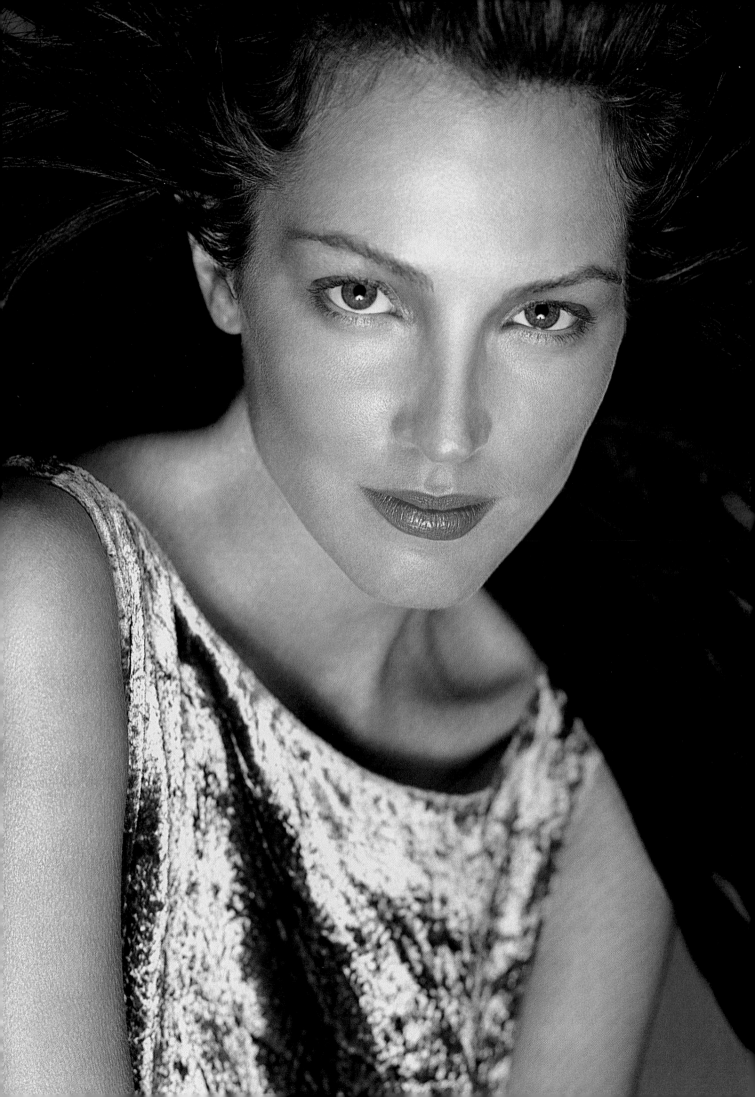

CHEEKS

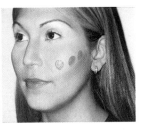

Blush Basics
Cream Blush Kevyn used cream formulas for a pretty, dewy look. Apply with your fingertip or a sponge, then blend.

Color Check
Kevyn loved pure, bright pigments. Don't be intimidated if blush looks very intense in the packaging. Bold shades are surprisingly beautiful when used with a light hand.

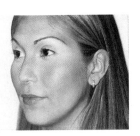

Liquid Blush Kevyn loved liquid formulas for a sheer, flushed finish. Apply with your fingertip or a sponge to moisturized skin. Blend immediately, because this type of blush sets very quickly. Wash your hands right away to avoid pink fingertips.

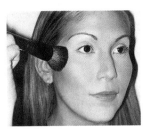

Powder Blush Great for all skin types, this blush blends and adheres best on a powdered face. Throw away the tiny brush that comes with your blush compact. It is impossible to get a natural-looking, even application with something so small. Apply instead with a large blush brush.

Get the Glow
• For a sweet, natural look, Kevyn applied blush to the apples of the cheeks (just smile to find yours) with his fingers or a brush.
• One of his favorite tricks for looking fresh-faced was to use cream blush, followed by translucent powder, and finished with powder blush.
• For a dramatic look, Kevyn contoured the face, then applied blush along the cheekbones, from the apples to the hairline.
• To warm the face and add a hint of contouring, Kevyn used basic blush on the temples, chin, and bridge of the nose.
• He liked to highlight the cheekbones for emphasis and added dimension. Use a shimmer cream on top of your cream blush or a reflective powder over your powder blush.

Kevyn's Favorite Tools • Large powder brush • Cream blush • Liquid blush
• Powder blush • Shimmer cream • Shimmer powder • Sponge

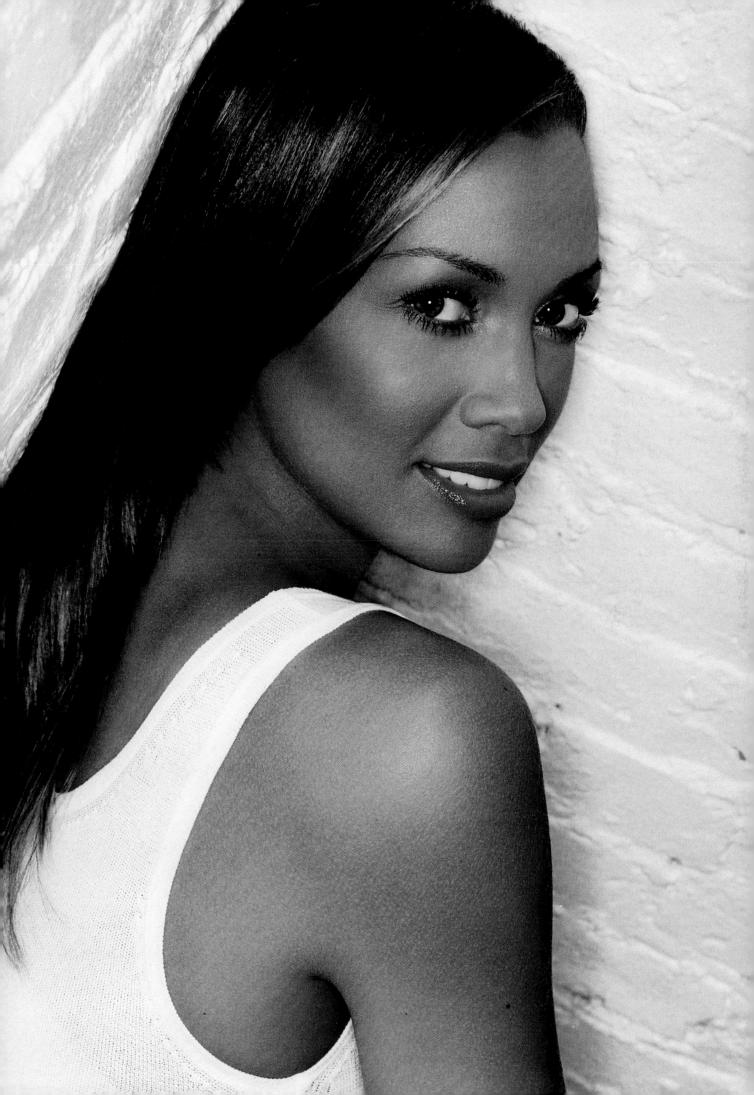

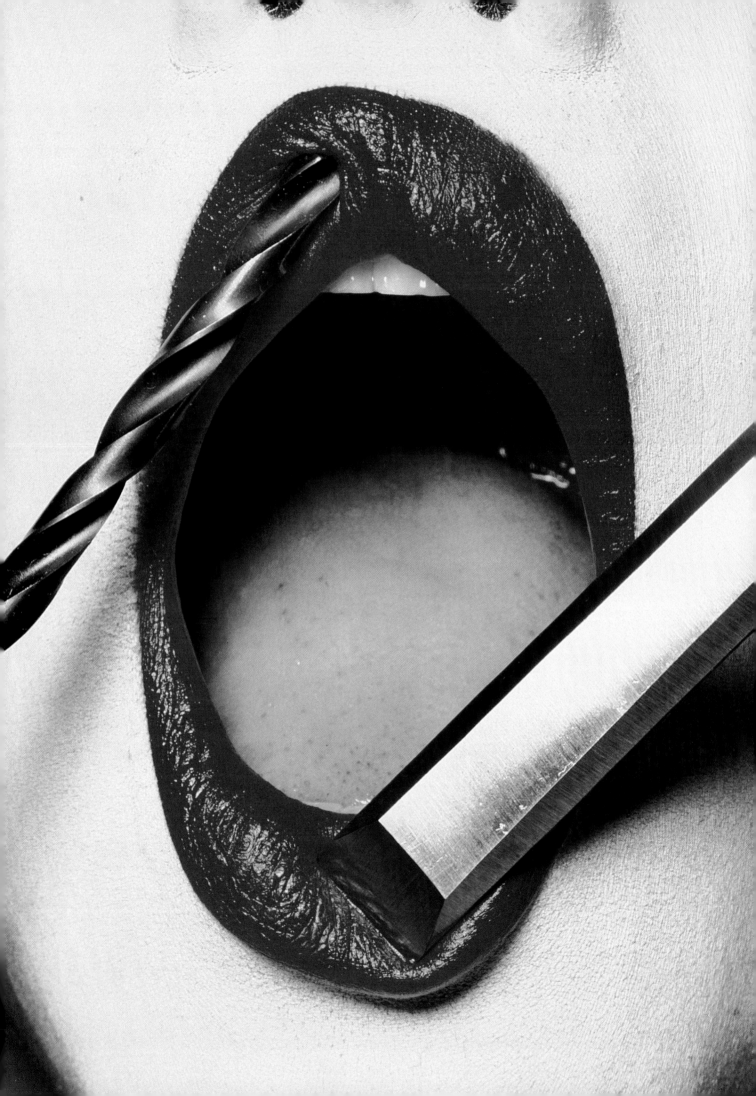

LIPS

"Watch that lip liner! Unless you know what you're doing, you're gonna look like trailer trash or a transvestite." **Tori Amos**

Getting Started Don't apply product to dry lips. If they're chapped, apply balm or petroleum jelly, then brush lightly with a toothbrush to get rid of any flaky skin. Use foundation or concealer to even out skin tone or discoloration.

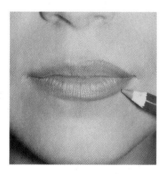 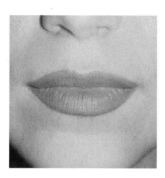

Shaping the Lip Kevyn used lip pencil to change or emphasize the shape of the mouth. Make your mouth appear larger, rounder, or more defined by outlining or drawing outside the lip line with a pencil that matches your lip color. Or make your lips smaller by drawing around the lip line with a flesh-colored pencil.

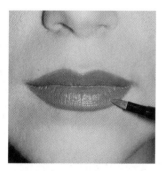

Lipstick That Lasts For a pout with staying power, Kevyn filled in the entire lip area with pencil, then applied a coat of lipstick with a lip brush and blotted with a tissue. (You'll get more control and a more precise application if you use a lip brush instead of applying straight from the tube.) Dust a thin layer of powder on the lips, then apply lipstick, and blot again.

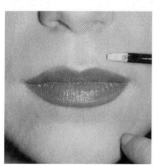

Sexy Pout To make lips appear more luscious, Kevyn added a little shimmer cream to the V right above the cupid's bow after applying lipstick. Then he put a dot of the shimmer cream on the center of the bottom lip and blended lightly. (You can also use pale shimmery gloss.)

kevyn aucoin: a beautiful life

The Three-Dimensional Lip Kevyn used this trick to create the appearance of full, pouty lips. It requires three colors from the same family: dark, medium, and light. The dark shade should be your lip liner and the medium shade your lipstick. For the light shade, you can use lipstick, lip gloss, or concealer.

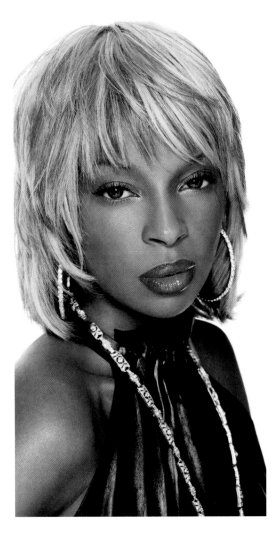

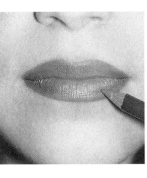

1. Prep your lips with a bit of balm. (Not too much, or lip color won't adhere.) Then line your lips, and fill in with the liner.

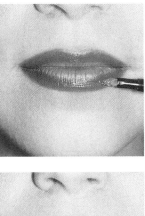

2. With a lip brush, apply lipstick inside the lip liner. Blend the lipstick into the lip liner, but don't erase the outside line. You want each layer of color to graduate into the next.

3. Dab the light color on the center of the upper and lower lips, and blend lightly with your finger.

The Red Lip "Kevyn loved this look," says Troy Surratt, the makeup artist who frequently assisted Kevyn on shoots. "He would paint it on with the utmost precision. It would be the sharpest, most perfect lip line you ever saw. He did it in one fell swoop, from corner to corner, with a lip brush." Kevyn then applied one coat of lipstick, blotted with a tissue, then applied again. If you want to change or define your lip shape, line and fill in with a lip-colored pencil first.

Kevyn's Favorite Tools • Lip brush • Lip balm • Lip liner • Lip gloss • Lipstick • Liquid shimmer cream • Translucent powder • Tissues

Opposite: Demi Moore by Matthew Rolston for Spanish *Vogue* © Condé Nast Publications Inc.

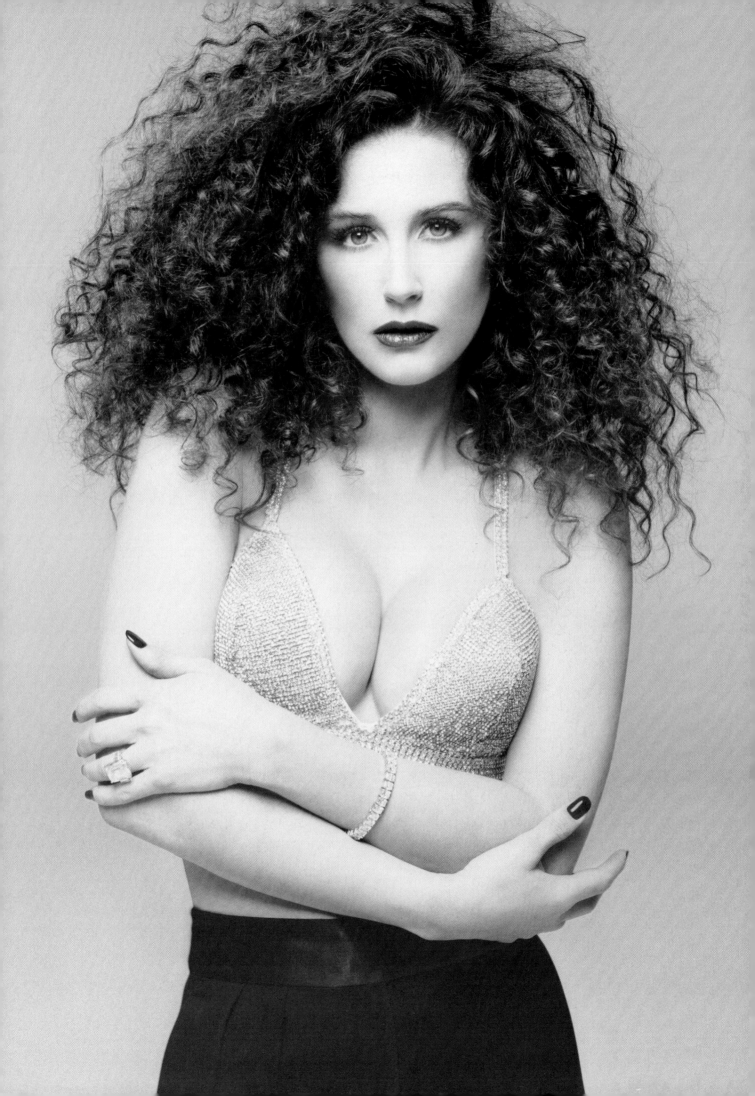

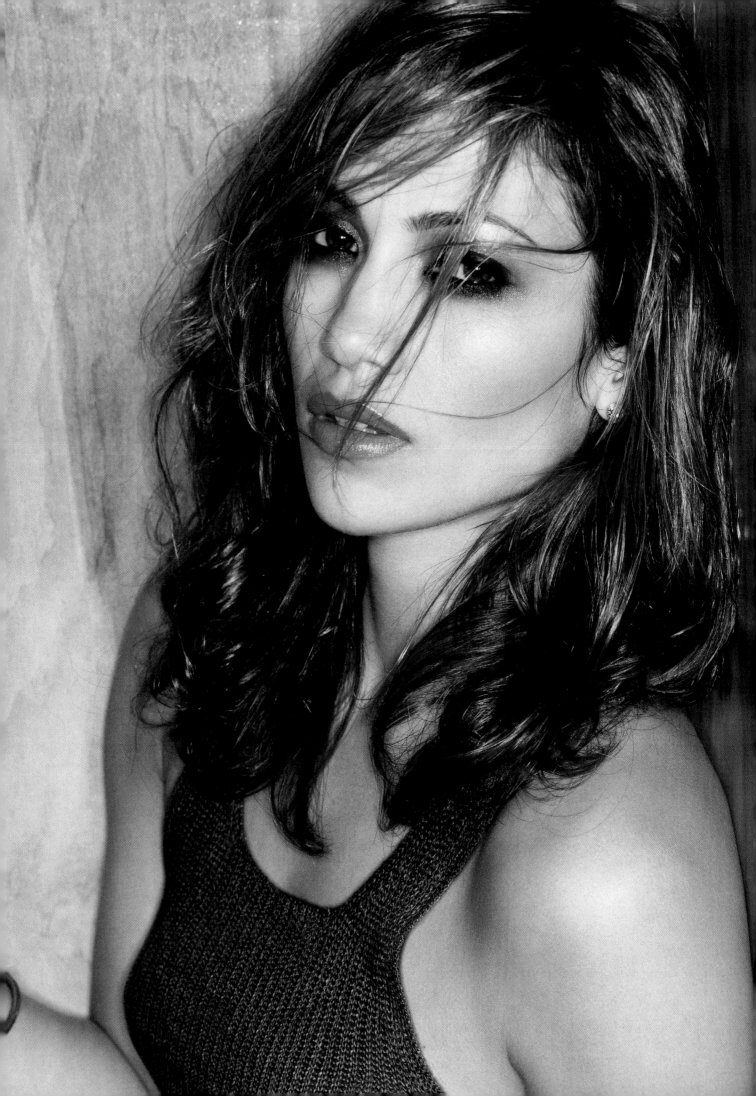

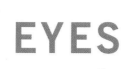

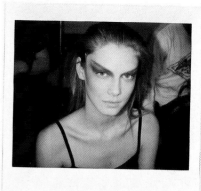

Opposite: Jennifer Lopez by Kevyn for *Marie Claire.*

EYES

"He always had a way of making eyes look doe-y, as in a deer. He'd sort of drag the eyeshadow out from the corners of the eye, and it would give you that effect. Now I do it a lot." **Jewel**

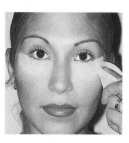

Powder Makes Perfect
When powdering the face, Kevyn put extra loose powder under the eyes. This allowed him to sweep away any excess product that fell there during eye makeup application. You also can use powder or cream-to-powder foundation to tone down eyeshadow if the color is too intense.

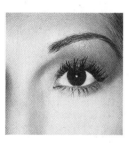

The Contoured Eye

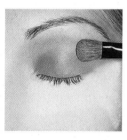

1. Brush a light-to-medium base color from lash line to brow with a medium eyeshadow brush.

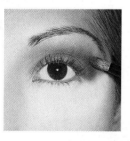

2. Starting at the outer corner of the eye, blend a darker color into the crease using a medium flat-tipped eyeshadow brush. Work from the outside in to prevent shadow from falling onto the cheeks or under the eye. Follow the crease until directly above the pupil. For a dramatic look, Kevyn followed the crease until it met the contouring along the sides of the nose.

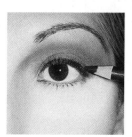

3. To finish, draw along the upper lash line with a soft dark pencil, then curl the lashes and apply mascara.

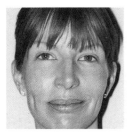

before

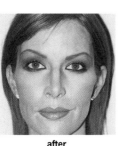

after

The Smoky Eye Although smoky implies black and gray shades, this look can be done in any color variation.

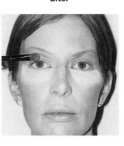

1. Apply a neutral base color to the entire eyelid, from lash line to brow bone.

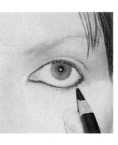

2. Line the inner rim of the entire eye with a dark eye pencil. Then, with the same pencil, line along the upper and lower lashes, getting right into the lash line so there are no discernible spaces.

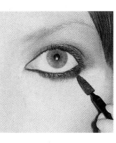

3. Smudge the liner with a sponge-tipped applicator. Then apply dark powder eyeshadow right over the pencil to set and soften.Using a medium shadow, encircle the eye around the outside of the dark liner/shadow. Blend into the dark circle around the eye, but don't erase the dark line. The goal here is to have a gradation of color. Curl lashes, and apply mascara.

Liner Know-How

• When using pencil eyeliner, get right into the lash line so there is no discernible space between the eyeliner and the lashes. Wiggle the pencil between the lashes to fill in any gaps.

• To apply liquid liner, Kevyn pulled the eyelid taut by lightly stretching it up and out. Then he drew a line as close to the lashes as possible. If you want to lift the eye, wing the line at the outer corner up slightly, not down.

• If you've never used liquid liner, line the upper lid with an eye pencil first, then trace over the line with liquid liner. If you're using a liquid with a brush applicator, wipe off excess product with a tissue.

• Women with small eyes and/or lines, dark circles, and puffiness around their eyes should skip liner underneath the eyes, suggested Kevyn.

• Line the inside lower rims of your eyes with white or beige eyeliner to make your eyes appear bigger and brighter.

kevyn aucoin: a beautiful life

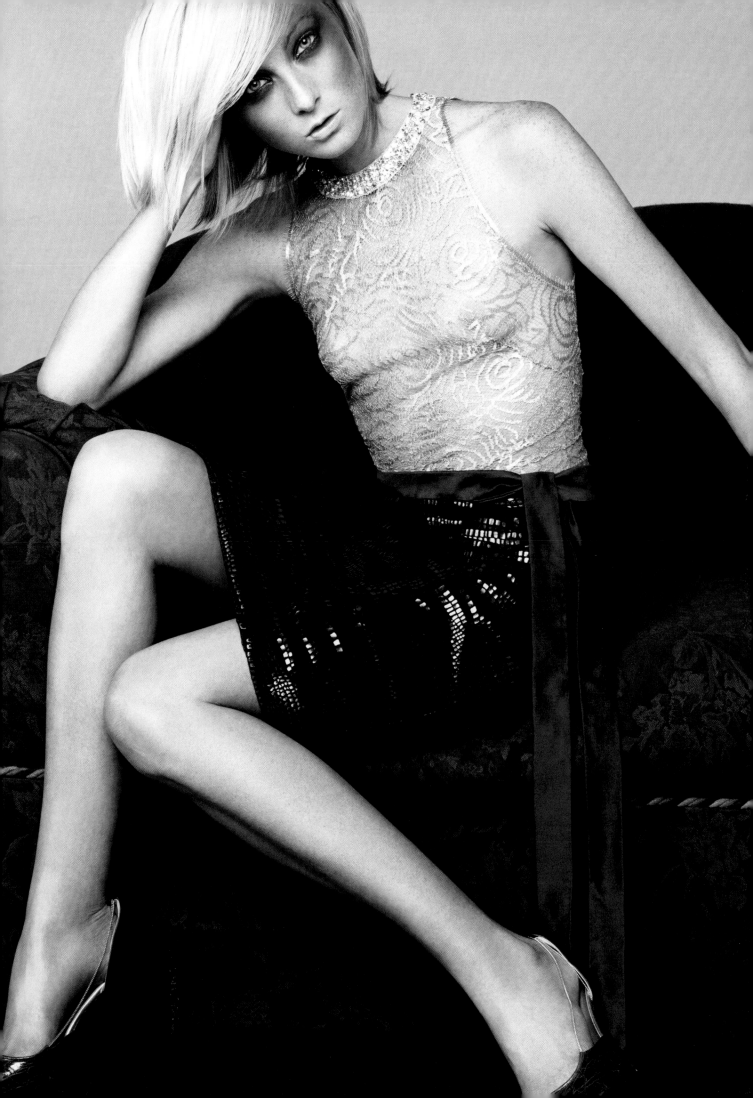

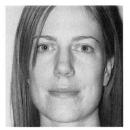

before

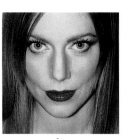

after

The Wide-Eyed Look Audrey Hepburn taught
Kevyn this trick for making the eyes appear wider-set.
The illusion helps pull attention outward by going from
light to dark, from the inner corner to the outer corner.

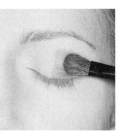

1. Apply a light base color to the entire lid and around the tear duct.

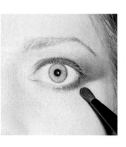

2. Apply a dark color along the crease from the pupils outward. Continue in a V shape to the side of the eye, beneath the bottom lashes, stopping at the pupil. You can pull the V out to the side as far as you wish. Just make sure to blend so there are no hard edges. Line your eyes if you wish. Finish by curling lashes and applying mascara.

Instant Radiance

One of Kevyn's signature tricks was highlighting the skin surrounding the tear ducts with a shimmery liquid, pencil, or eyeshadow. He would follow the natural V shape, then blend with a small brush or his finger. This trick was inspired by Kevyn's niece Falon. When she was born, Kevyn couldn't help but notice how the skin around her eyes just glistened.

Kevyn also would put shimmer cream directly on the brow bone, underneath the brows, to make the eyes look bigger and more luminous and to draw attention to a nicely arched eyebrow.

Kevyn's Favorite Tools • Powder eyeshadow • Cream eyeshadow • Pencil eyeliner
• Liquid eyeliner • Liquid shimmer cream • Medium brush • White or beige eyeliner • Sponge

Opposite: Britney by Steven Klein for her *Britney* CD.

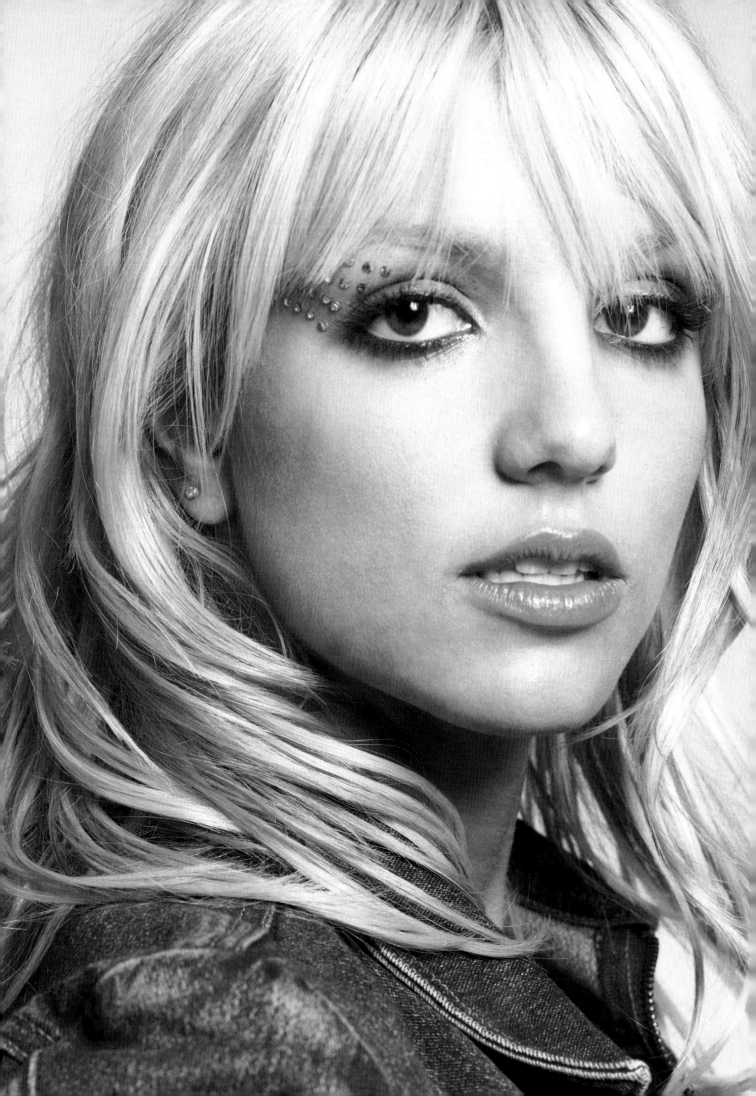

"Kevyn and I were always on the same wavelength. I could just say, 'I. Eyelashes. Think. Christy.' And he was like, 'Got it!'" **Isaac Mizrahi**

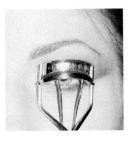

Curling Made Simple "Curling your lashes opens your eyes and makes you look brighter, younger, and fresher," said Kevyn about one of his favorite tricks. Start at the very base of the lashes, and press firmly. Don't pull at the lashes or pinch the skin; that's how you'll lose precious hairs. (Fact: They do grow back.) If necessary, move the curler to the middle of the lashes, and crimp again; then move further out, and repeat. Kevyn referred to this as "pumping and walking out." This prevents your lashes from curling at a right angle. Don't apply mascara until you're finished.

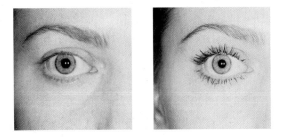

Lush and Long Kevyn liked mascara wands with a small applicator brush because that allowed him to get as close as possible to the lash line. Kevyn applied as many coats of mascara as needed. He liked to wipe the wand on a tissue in between coats to remove excess product (again, use the cheap kind; super-soft ones will leave fuzz behind). "I like the base of the lashes to have more product, with the ends being fine and lengthened," he said. Kevyn would brush out the mascara with a lash comb. This helps to "unclump" the lashes.

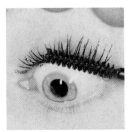

1. Hold the applicator horizontally, wiggle it into the very base of the lashes, then sweep along the length of the lashes.

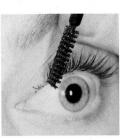

2. Hold the brush vertically and go lash by lash.

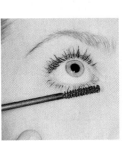

3. Wiggle along the bottom lashes.

Opposite: Celine Dion by Kevyn for *Marie Claire*.

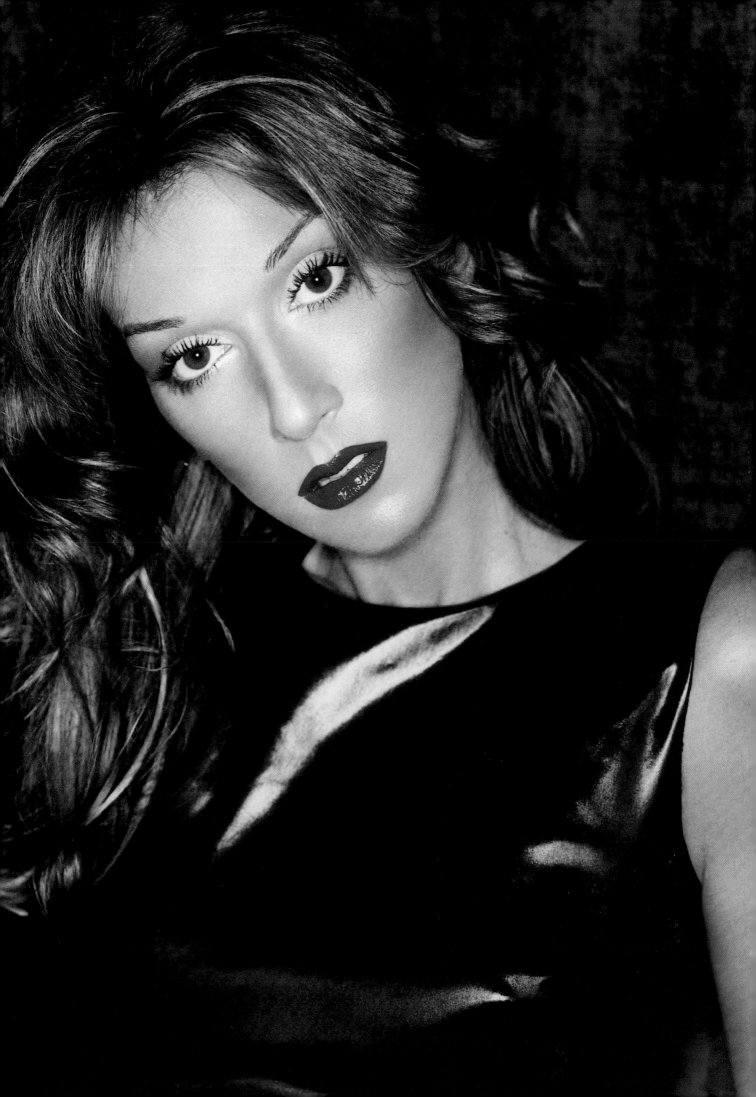

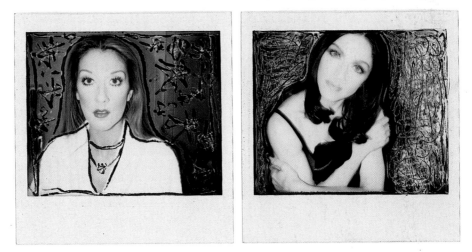

Low-maintenance Lashes
Kevyn recommended that his fair-haired friends get their lashes tinted black at a salon. This turns the blondest, barely there lashes inky black. You can just curl your lashes and go. No mascara necessary.

Colored Mascara
Don't be afraid to go beyond basic black and brown. Kevyn loved how red and burgundy mascara played against different eye colors. Some colored mascaras are thicker than regular ones, but these heavier formulas can really build up the lashes. Just pump the brush into the tube, and apply as many coats as necessary.

Faking It
For Kevyn, nothing added oomph to a face like false eyelashes. He preferred strip lashes with a clear- or natural-colored band instead of a black one. "If the strip is longer than the length of your lash line, you can trim it," he said. "If you find a pair that doesn't look natural, take nail scissors, and trim every other lash so they're all different lengths. Apply glue to the lash strip, hold it in front of you until the glue is tacky (otherwise it'll slide all over your eyes), then place the strip as close to your natural lashes as possible. (The back end of a pair of tweezers can often help push a lash down.)"

Gena Rowlands taught Kevyn a goof-proof trick for the most accurate application. Match the center of the lash strip with the center of the lash line, then firmly press the ends down.

Once the glue is dry, curl all the lashes together. Apply mascara to your real lashes and the false ones. Mascara also helps cover any obvious glue.

For a more natural look, you can use a few individual lashes to boost your lash line. Follow the same directions as above.

Kevyn's Favorite Tools • Black mascara • Dark red/burgundy mascara • Lash curler
• Lash comb/separator • False lashes (individual and strip) • Lash glue

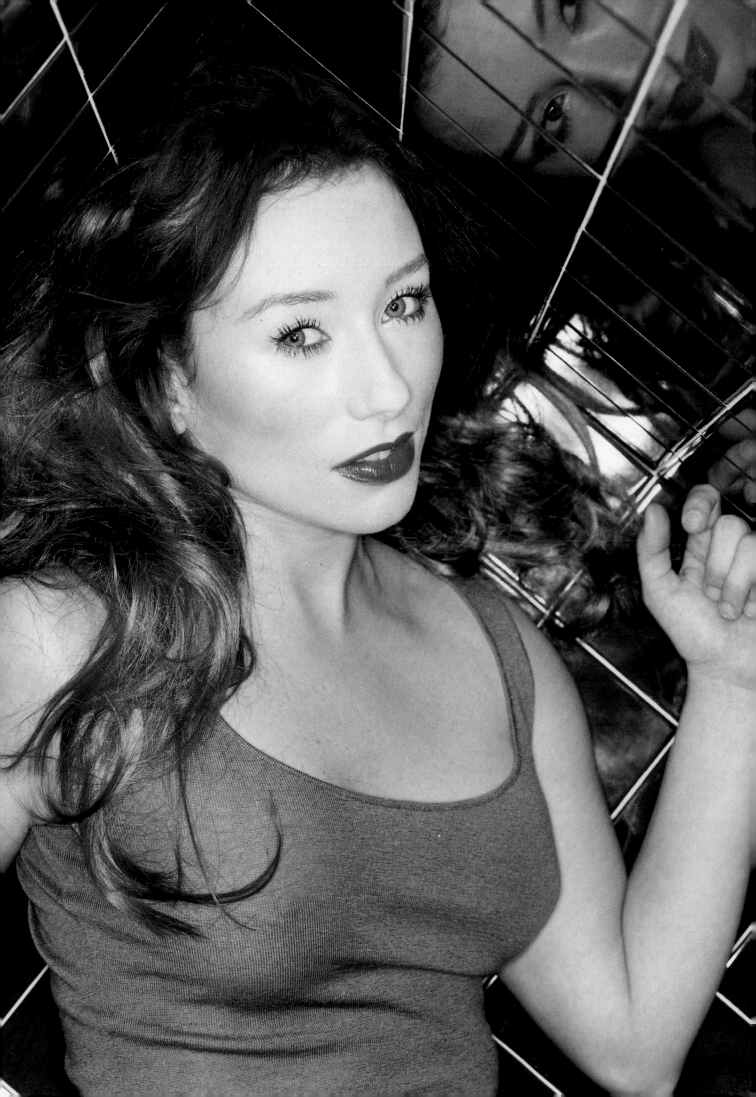

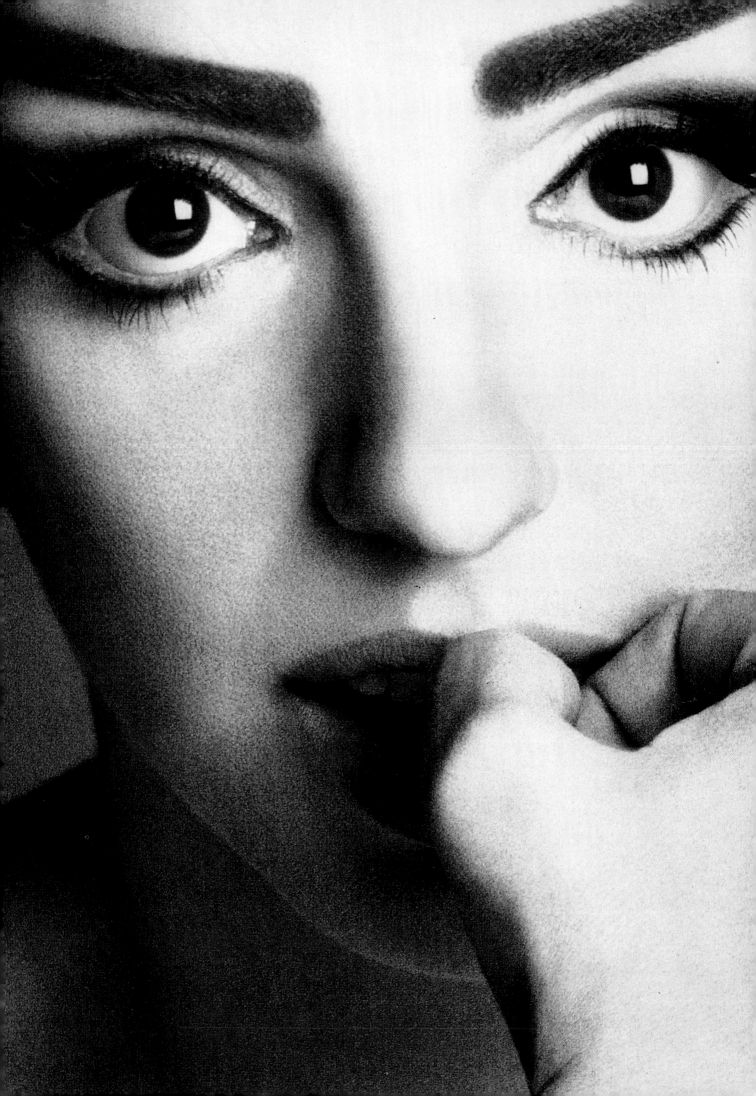

Opposite: Liza by Steven Meisel © 1990 Italian *Vogue*. Courtesy of Condé Nast Publications Inc.

BROWS

before

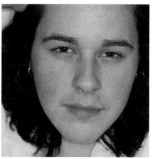

Perfect Arches Every Time

Don't be afraid to do your own brows. It's easier than you think. This method lets you design the shape before tweezing. The goal here is to clean up and define your brows. As Kevyn always said, the most dramatic thing you can do to change your look is to shape your eyebrows. Just don't try this on the day of a big event. Pick a time when you can concentrate.

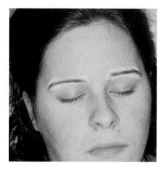

1. Take a white eyeliner or concealer pencil, and draw above and below the brow to achieve the shape you want. Draw right over the hairs that should be tweezed. Step back and see if you like the shape.

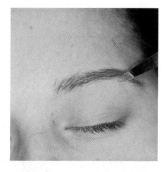

2. Tweeze one hair at a time, following the shape that you have drawn. Remember, it's better to undertweeze. (If you tweeze too much, skip ahead for advice on penciling in your brows.) Kevyn would use wax strips to remove the fine hairs under and between the brows and between the ends of the brows and the hairline. If you have long brow hairs, trim rather than tweeze. Brush them upward with a brow brush or toothbrush, then cut with nail scissors. It's easy to cut them too short, so be careful.

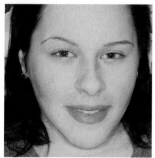

after

Penciling In

Kevyn preferred pencil instead of powder when it came to filling in sparse brows or drawing a new brow shape. He suggested that brunettes and redheads choose a shade lighter than their natural brow color. Blondes should go for a slightly darker shade. Make sure the pencil is sharp, and use light, feathery strokes for the most natural results. Kevyn finished the look with some brow gel to keep the hairs in place.

Brow Wow

For extra drama, highlight your brows. Kevyn used a bit of gold mascara in place of brow gel, or he mixed a bit of gold eyeshadow or powder with hair wax or pomade and brushed it through the brows.

kevyn aucoin: a beautiful life

227

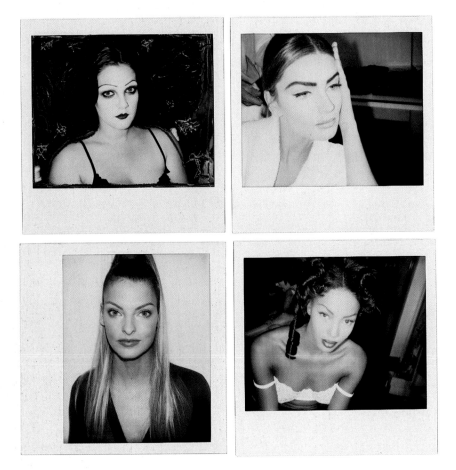

"When Kevyn does my face, I don't even have to look in the mirror. He knows all its secrets. . . .
He knows I don't like my eyebrows too tweezed," **said Cindy Crawford.**
"But tweezing your eyebrows can change your entire face. It can change everything," **said Kevyn.**
"It can make you a better person," **Cindy replied.**

Boost Your Brow Color

Kevyn loved to lighten the brows for a soft but modern look. He mixed a small batch of cream bleach, applied it to the brows, and checked the color every few minutes. (Be very cautious when using bleach around your eyes. Do a test patch on your skin first to make sure you don't have a negative reaction to the product.) When he achieved the desired shade, he rinsed the product away according to the directions on the box. If you'd rather darken your brows, you can do this with a pencil, or you can have them tinted at a salon.

Kevyn's Favorite Tools • Sharp tweezers • White eyeliner • Eyebrow pencil • Cotton swabs • Cream bleach • Brow brush • Brow grooming gel • Nail scissors

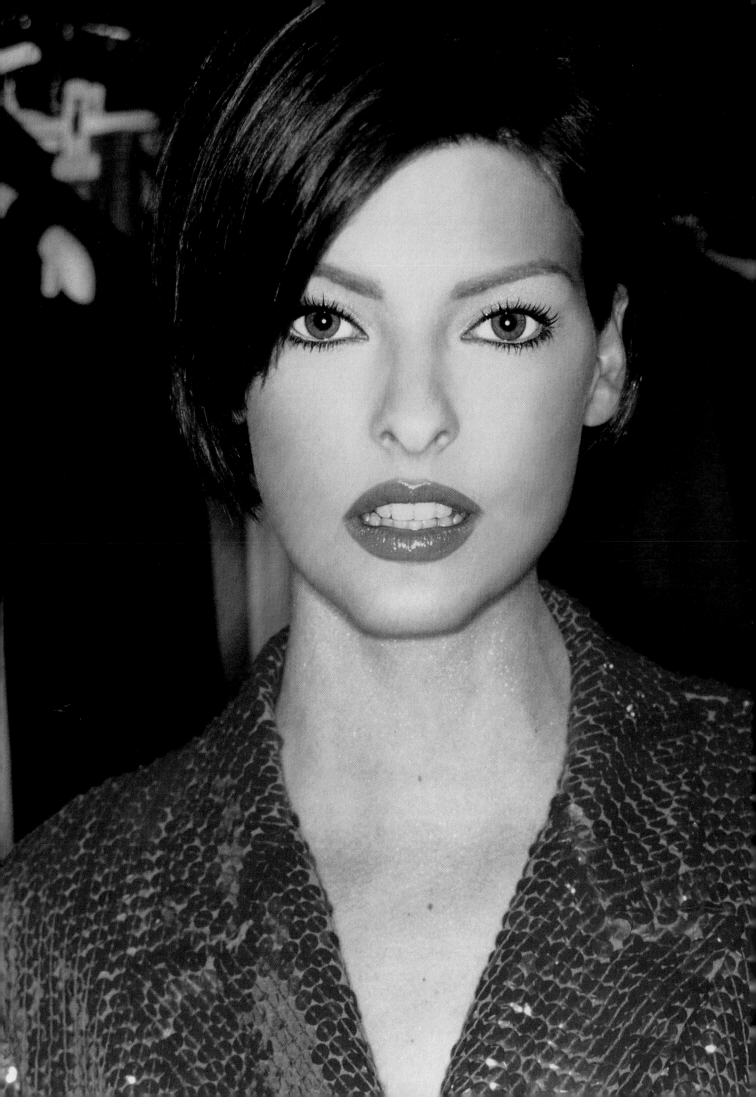

AFTERWORD BY SAMANTHA ADKISSON

Kevyn was my best friend, my angel, my hero, my inspiration, my teacher, my dad, and my uncle. He was always there for me no matter what I did. He taught me everything I know about feelings, love, and art. He always introduced me to the prettiest music, the best movies, the most beautiful paintings. He was the most memorable person in my life. I always imagined him flying down to Louisiana for my prom, to do my makeup and share that moment with me. I always pictured him there for my wedding day, to walk me down the aisle along with my father.

He ranked among the most beautiful people in my life. I don't mean physically beautiful, even though he was. When I looked deep into his soul, I could see that he was the most beautiful person around. He was the reason I started writing poetry. He was the reason I believed in myself.

Kevyn gave me things not many other people get to have. He gave me a wonderful life, lots of love, and beauty. He gave me beauty above all things. I am not a beautiful person on the outside, and not so much on the inside, but he tried to make me beautiful all the way through. He also taught me to recognize beauty in everyone I meet.

I miss him terribly, but I know he is still with me—guiding me and teaching me. Kevyn gave me a card a few years ago that starts by saying "I'm on your side, and I always will be," and he is. Kevyn always said the song "The Horses" by Rickie Lee Jones was our song and I think he was right. "We'll be riding on the horses, yea, way up in the sky, little darlin', and if you fall I'll pick you up . . ." He always picks me up when I fall. And I fall a lot so he must be a pretty busy angel.

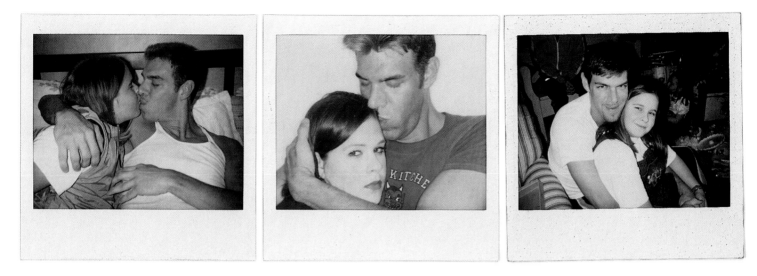

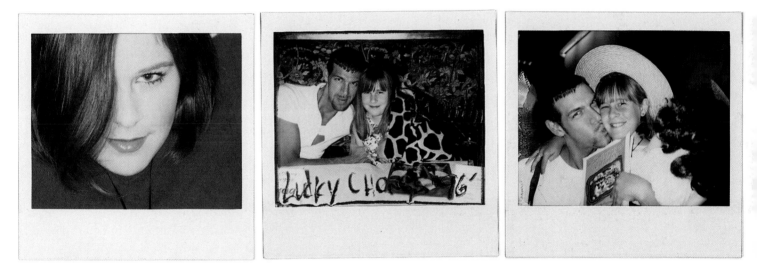

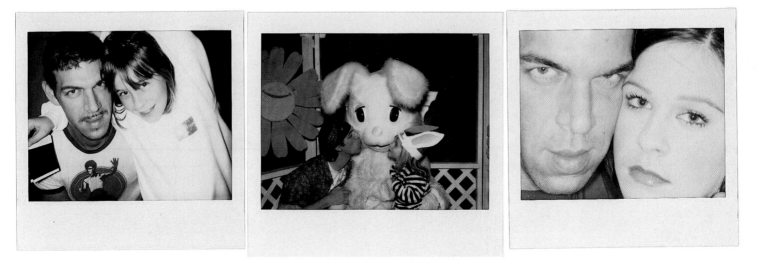

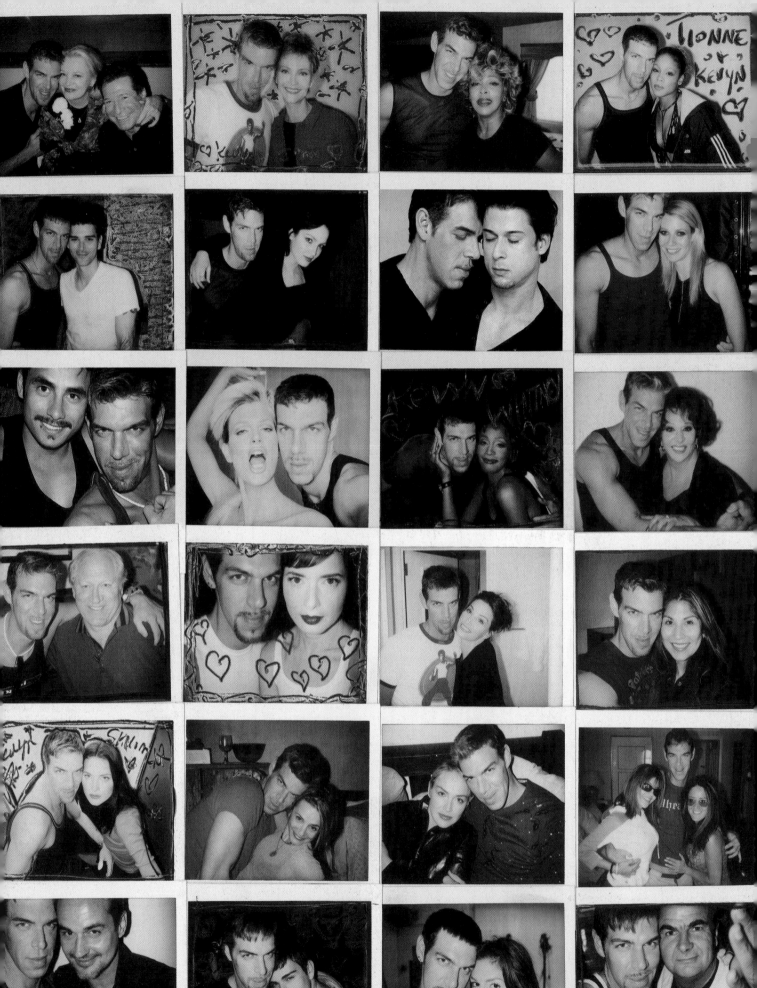

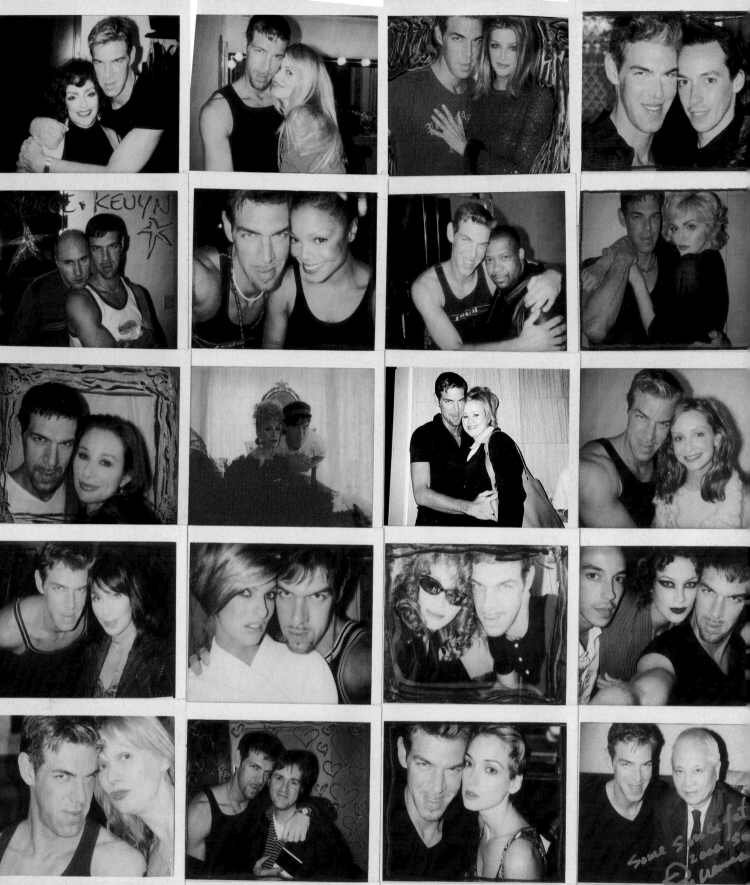

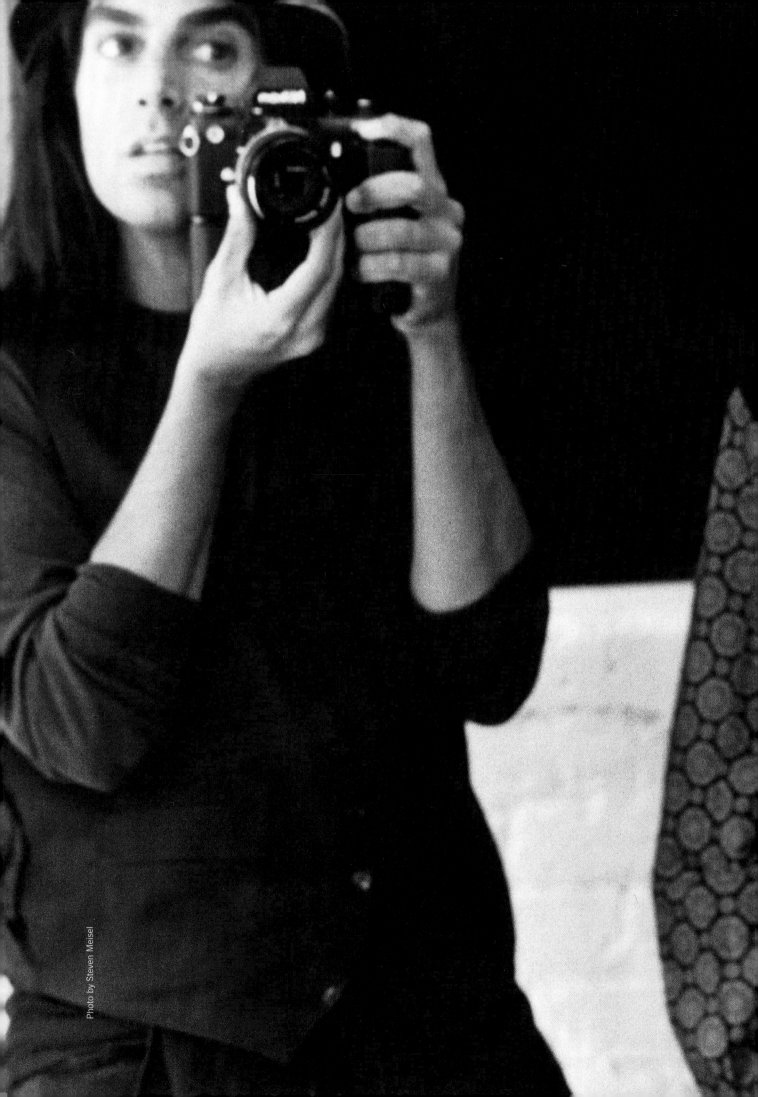

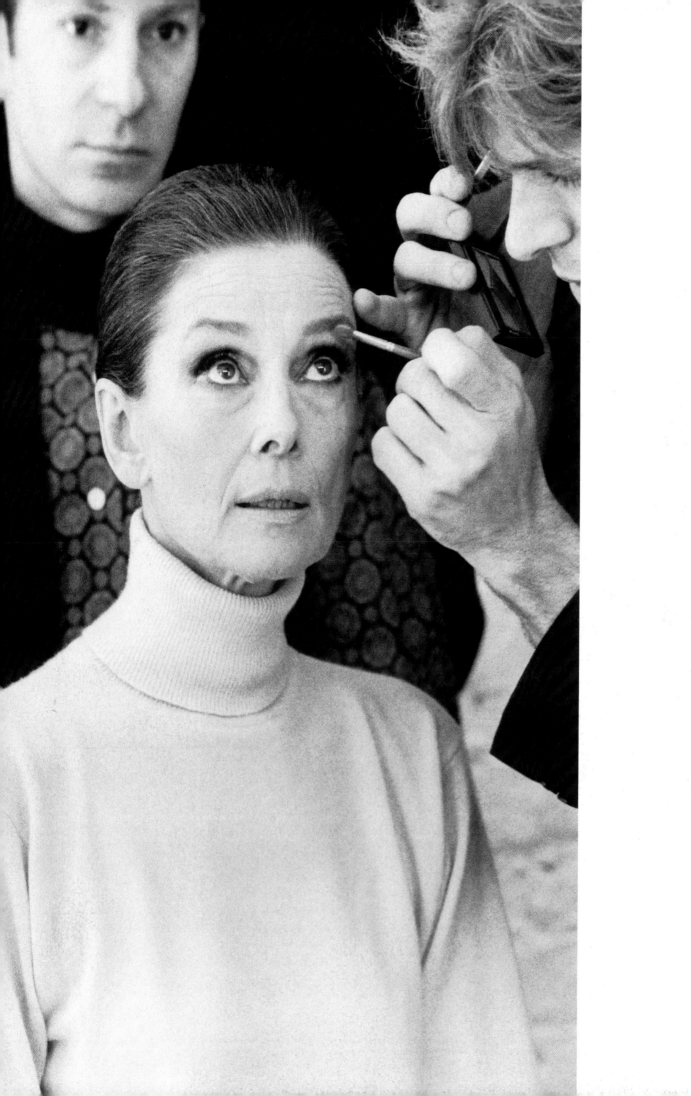

pp. 232 & 233 - Friends collage:

First row, Kevyn with Gena Rowlands and Robert Forrest; Joan Allen; Tina Turner; Tionne "T-Boz" Watkins; Liza Minnelli; Claudia Schiffer; Kirstie Alley; and Orlando Pita. Second row: Tom Woolley; Chandra North; Todd Littleton; Gwyneth Paltrow; Serge Normant; Janet Jackson; Kithe Brewster; and Sophie Dahl. Third row: Thomas Efaw; Kristen McMenamy; Whitney Houston; Sylvia Browne; Tori Amos; Joan Rivers; Caroline Rhea; and Calista Flockhart. Fourth row: Jerry Burch; Isabella Rossellini; Gina Gershon; Sandra Collado; Cher; Linda Evangelista; Julia Roberts; Orlando Pita and Carolyn Murphy. Fifth row: Shalom Harlow; Amy Sedaris; Sharon Stone; Julie Mijares and Dee Ragano; Eveline Lange; Robert Montgomery; Winona Ryder; and Shu Uemura. Sixth row: Oribe; Rubin Singer; Cindy Crawford; Patrick Demarchelier; Jewel; Alex Perruzzi; Dido; and Lisa Marie Presley.